COMMONSENSE CHILDREARING

Commonsense Childrearing

Unconventional Wisdom for a Nourished Childhood

Thomas Cowan, MD

SteinerBooks | 2025

2025
SteinerBooks
An imprint of Anthroposophic Press, Inc.
834 Main Street, PO Box 358
Spencertown, New York 12165
www.steinerbooks.org

Cover design by Lance Buckley

LIBRARY OF CONGRESS CONTROL NUMBER: 2024946384

ISBN: 978-1-938685-57-6

Printed in the United States of America
by Versa Press, Inc.

Contents

Part I

1.   Choosing Sides   3
2.   Trust   10
3.   Rhythm   16
4.   Perseverance   24
5.   Play   34
6.   Integrity   42
7.   Food Fights   50
8.   Punishments and Rewards   56

Part II

9.   School   73
10.   Radical Monopolies: The Hidden Curriculum   83
11.   Education   93
12.   Learning to Read   106
13.   Electronic Devices   113
14.   Returning to Life   120
15.   Envisioning a World Fit for Our Children   128
16.   Vaccines and Animals   134

Appendices:

    1. Electromagnetic Frequencies   141
    2. Tylenol   146
    3. Diagnostic Ultrasounds   152

Bibliography   157
Index   159

Part I

CHAPTER ONE

Choosing Sides

About eighteen years ago, I had an experience that forever changed my views on raising children. It wasn't as if it came out of the blue, as my views had certainly been moving in that direction for years before that. But it was one of those galvanizing events that, however small it seemed at the time, changed my views for good. There was no going back.

In medicine, it is a kind of cliché for doctors to say they learn many important things from their patients. We heard it often in medical school and residency, and it continues in one's further medical education. In contrast, what I frequently hear from my patients is they did something unusual for whatever ails them, they excitedly went to tell their doctor about it, and the doctor was either not interested or outright dismissive. I have made it my practice for decades that if a patient comes in and tells me they cured their lupus by drinking horse urine, I ask them how much and which horse. It's not necessarily that I automatically believe that this intervention actually cured their lupus or that it will be a therapy worth me looking into, but as a matter of respect for the patient, I owe it to them to listen. Also, I can categorically state that many, if not most of the successful therapies I have used in my career as a doctor have first been brought to me by my patients. The key, though, is knowing how to ask, how to listen, and how to put this into a larger framework. That is the "technique" of learning from patients—a skill most doctors are sorely lacking.

Let me set the stage for my experience of eighteen years ago, in which a seven-year-old boy taught me a life-changing lesson. In some ways, this book is a way of thanking that guy for taking the trouble to be straight up with me and trusting that I would listen.

At the time, I had been a doctor for about twenty years. For most of those twenty years, I had been practicing anthroposophical medicine in my small general practice. I was also the school doctor for three different Waldorf schools. From the early days of the Waldorf school movement in the 1920s, the college of teachers would meet once a month with the school doctor to have a "child study." In a child study, the various teachers of the child would present their observations and their picture of the child to the entire faculty. In addition, the school doctor would examine the child in their office and observe the child for a two-hour period one morning. Then the school doctor would add their observations to the developing picture of the child presented at the child study. The purpose of the child study was not necessarily to "fix" the child as much as to gain a fuller understanding of just who this human being is.

Having done this for three different schools for twenty years, once per month with each school, I had built up significant experience with observing children, working with children in need, and observing various teachers. Over that time, I seemed to develop at least some skill in presenting imaginative pictures of children, which helped the teachers work with that child in the future. The experience I had eighteen years ago happened when a nearby Waldorf school, which had no trained doctor in their community, asked me to come down for two days to observe various children in their school and to do a number of child studies for the children I had observed. This two-day visit also came about six months after my first exposure to nonviolent communication (NVC), which influenced the way I conducted my interviews and examinations of the children. In those six months, I intensively studied the work of Carl Rogers—the man Marshall Rosenberg talked about as being the inspiration for NVC—in particular the way he conducted interviews. This is the brief background for the meeting with my seven-year-old friend.

As I set up to work that day in a school I had never visited before, I established the "rules" of how I wanted to conduct my day. The school wanted me to see children they were having issues with, either in relation to behavior or learning, or sometimes physical health challenges. The parents had all consented to my seeing the child one time as a "patient." I asked the primary teacher of the child to write no more than one paragraph explaining why they wanted me to see the child. Then I explained to the parent(s) and child, as they sat down in the exam room, that the first thing I did in these exams was speak directly and ask questions directly to the child. I asked that the parents not intervene or interrupt, no matter how much they disagreed with the child or even if they thought the child was giving me factually inaccurate information. No matter what, no interruptions. Once I had finished talking to the child, I would give the parent(s) whatever time they needed to tell me whatever they wanted to say. They could fill in details, correct things the child said, or whatever. However, in this phase, I asked that the child be allowed to interrupt the parent. I usually said I realized this was not "fair" but these are the "rules." In all cases, the parents agreed to these rules.

I don't remember much about this particular boy's appearance, only that he appeared robust and had a baseball cap pulled down over his eyes. I explained the "rules" and the mother agreed and only said he probably won't talk to you much. I read the paragraph written by his first-grade teacher, which told me he had no particular physical complaints but was very disruptive in class, even physically lashing out at other children, to the point that they didn't know if they could allow him to continue at the school. As the parents were dedicated to the Waldorf ideals, this was a real crisis for the school and the family. What follows below is my paraphrased recollection of the important points of our dialogue. Obviously, I don't remember his exact words, but the gist of it is accurate.

> Me: Hey, how's it going?
> Boy: Ok.
> Me: I hear you're in first grade, is that correct?
> Boy: Yes.
> Me: How's it going in school?
> Boy: Fine.

At this point, I probably asked a few more general questions about how many brothers and sisters he had, what he likes to do, things like that. In each case, he would give one-word answers, clearly not that interested in talking much to me. At some point, soon, I got back to the issue:

Me: So, I hear there are some troubles at school,
       do you know anything about this?
Boy: Yes, my teacher lies.

The mother was clearly taken aback and looked like she wanted to say something, I gave her a look as if to remind her of the "rules," and she remained quiet. The important step at this point is to continue the dialogue and get as much information as possible but never to ask a "why" question. For some reason, that seems to stop the dialogue in its tracks and leads nowhere.

Me: What does she lie about?
Boy: Well, the other day she said I hit Freddy, but I
       didn't, and the teacher said I did and lied about it.
Me: Can you tell me what happened that led up to her
       saying you hit Freddy
Boy: Freddy shot a spit ball at my friend Joey. I told
       Freddy to stop and he wouldn't.
Me: Then what happened?
Boy: I kept telling him to stop and he wouldn't listen.
       Another boy laughed at Joey and called him a
       baby.
Me: Then what did you do?
Boy: I went over to Freddy and said he had to stop
       now, but he wouldn't listen. He pushed me so I
       pushed him back, and that was the end of it. The
       teacher saw me push Freddy and sent me out of
       the room. She lied. Freddy pushed me first. She
       always lies and blames me for everything.
Me: Can you think of another time when she blamed
       you for something?
Boy: Yes, it happens almost every day; someone
       laughs or talks loud, and so I join in the laughing.
       She only punishes me. It's not fair.

Me: Was there something that happened the other
    day?

Boy: Yes, she lied again, someone threw a glass at one
    of the other kids, not me, and the teacher blamed
    me for it. She lies all the time.

Me: So you didn't throw the glass?

Boy: No, someone else did, but I would throw a glass.

Mother (who can't help herself): But the teacher said
    she saw you throw the glass. That's why you got
    sent home from school that day; someone could
    have gotten really hurt.

I reminded the mother of the rules, but since this was said, I
had to deal with it.

Me: Did you also throw a glass?

Boy: Jimmy threw the glass first, then other people
    threw things, and I threw a glass jar and it broke.

Me: Is there anything else about school you want to
    tell me?

At this point, the boy who supposedly wouldn't talk to me
launched into a ten-minute monologue about all the unfair
things that happened at school, how he was not allowed
to go out for recess—the only part he liked—if the class
was bad, how everyone talked out of turn, but the teacher
lied and blamed it on him. He talked about how he hated
school and wanted to play in the creek in the back of the
new house they had just moved into. Throughout this time,
I just kept asking him clarifying questions, mostly telling
him I just wanted to make sure I got the story correct. He
probably went on for half an hour describing everything in
life and school, and in particular everything that he thought
was unfair.

Mostly because I had other children to see, I said I needed to move on here but wanted to know if he thought I had heard his story and if he thought I understood the situation. He looked at his mother and said the first of two things that changed my world. He said, "Hey, he's on my side." At that point, you are allowed to ask one "why" question, only one, so make it a good one. I asked him, "So, why did you throw that glass jar?"

He looked at me and said, "So they would send me home and I would never come back."

I asked him my final question, which was: "Is there anything you would like me to do for you right now?"

He answered, "Yes, tell them to let me stay home and play or to stop lying."

I said I would do my best, but the outcome was probably not up to me. I asked the mother if she had anything she wanted to add, but she was too shaken up to say much. I examined him and told them both I would be talking to the teachers later that day. We shook hands, he gave me a big grin, and we parted ways.

Here is my first and most important message of this book, one that seems so simple but can be so hard to see. It is the message that came through loud and clear in this visit: If you want to raise a healthy child in a toxic culture, get on your child's side and stay there, *no matter what*.

The rest of the book explores what staying on your child's side really means.

CHAPTER TWO

Trust

Yes, yes, yes, I know. I can almost hear the chorus of parents, teachers, and pediatricians standing up and yelling: Don't you understand that what that boy did was unacceptable?! Someone could have been hurt by the broken glass; he needs to be helped to not have violent outbursts. Besides which, if he is disruptive in class and gets sent home, he won't learn to read, he won't get a good education, he'll never get into college, he'll never get a good job, and he may very well end up in prison. It's also possible he may have a diagnosable mental health condition called oppositional-defiance disorder for which he needs urgent treatment if he is to be successful in life, and—as my five-year-old grandson, Sam, apparently said to his pre-school teacher when confronted with his own "bad" behavior—bwah, bwah, bwah (Sam has trouble with his L's these days).

First of all, I want to point out that I didn't necessarily condone his throwing of the glass jar. I simply heard his story. His story made it clear that this action, and probably many others, were deliberate attempts to get thrown out of a school he clearly detested. If nothing else, one has to admire his cleverness and ingenuity. The next crucial point in his story, which came out in the twenty or so minutes in which he described his life, was that what he enjoyed most was going to the creek on his property with a bunch of his friends and catching tadpoles, watching snakes, fishing for whatever creatures they could find, building forts, and probably picking berries and other wild foods. He seemed to know a lot about these things, and when I asked him if he had any trouble getting along with his friends in his woods, he hardly knew what I was asking. "We just play," he said. My guess is that sometimes they fought, but mostly they were busy figuring out how to build the best fort and catch the biggest tadpole. My friend was learning a lot, which brings up perhaps the central question of this book: What do I mean by having success in raising a child? In other words, if we are to be successful in raising children, we need to put some attention on the difficult question of what our goal is here. That is, what does this "successfully" raised child look like?

Answering the question of the goal of raising a child is fraught with pitfalls. Children come into the world with their own destinies, their own strengths, weaknesses, dreams, and fears.

There is not one goal for all children; there is not one outcome that we are striving for.

However, there are some principles that I believe we can use to help guide our actions. For one, if the goal is to raise healthy children in a toxic world, then obviously our children must be physically healthy. No chronic diseases, no allergies, no prescription meds—none of that stuff, which is at epidemic levels in our children today. Without a level of robust health—mostly achievable through the guidelines I have outlined in previous books—we have a weak foundation on which to build. All children should eat a Nourishing

Traditions type of diet, eschew vaccinations, ultrasounds in pregnancy, and all the other routine interventions so common in today's world. For more information on the rationale for this, please consult *The Nourishing Traditions Book of Baby and Child Care,* as well as *Vaccines, Autoimmunity, and the Changing Nature of Childhood Illness.*

This book is concerned with the other aspects of raising a healthy child, which in many ways are just as important as the more "physical" interventions.

Again, knowing the difficulty of defining a "successful" person, we can draw on some of the luminaries in the fields of philosophy and child development to get a sense of what we mean by a healthy child. Here are a couple of my favorites:

> "Our highest endeavor must be to develop free human beings who are able of themselves to impart purpose and direction to their lives." —Rudolf Steiner

> "As soon as you trust yourself, you will know how to live." —Johann Wolfgang von Goethe

Free human beings, human beings who trust themselves, human beings who are happy, independent, and seek their unique destiny. Human beings who think deeply, who actively seek to understand how they and humanity in general fit into the larger world. Human beings who seek wisdom, justice, and compassion. Human beings who can love and be loved. Human beings who at the time of their death can look back on their lives without regret. Those are some of the qualities of a human being encompassed by the word "healthy." These qualities, and many others besides, should and must be the goal of our attempts to raise healthy children. These are also the qualities that are sorely lacking in humanity today. We have created, consciously or unconsciously, human beings who suffer from chronic poor health, who blindly believe what they are told or taught, who have an uncomfortable sense that something fundamental is not right with the world or with their place in the world or both. Human beings who can neither accept nor give love and whose interest in justice, wisdom, and compassion starts and ends with following causes on Facebook or posting a few tweets. The consequence of generations of human beings who have lost their way is that we face unprecedented catastrophes on so many fronts it is hard to keep track of them all. We have poisoned every inch of the only home we have and done so in the blink of an eye. We urgently need an answer to the question of what it takes to raise children so that they become adults who could never even consider destroying the only place they can call home. Are you really convinced that getting my little seven-year-old friend to be obedient in school, any school, or to be put on medication for his oppositional mental health disorder—as opposed to having him spend his days (for now) catching crawdads in the creek—will produce the type of human being we need so urgently these days? I, personally, am not convinced. We need, rather, to take a deep dive into the world of children and in particular try to understand how they learn.

Before we do that, I want to present what I think is the stark contrast between the type of free, courageous, independent human being who understands his own destiny and lives it to the fullest and the modern human being who does what he is told. To be clear, free and healthy human beings who trust in themselves will make moral judgments based on their own unique, personal experience and not on the morals of the culture they live in.

Heaven knows, the morals of the culture we live in have not just permitted but exalted a way of life that has led us to the brink of catastrophe. In the late 1960s, the U.S. was mired in one of a seemingly endless series of immoral and catastrophic wars, this time in Vietnam. The government was forcing all young men, whether they agreed or not, to be conscripted into the military and to go off to fight a war that was being fought for the flimsiest of reasons. In the face of this travesty, Muhammad Ali, the boxer, famously and courageously risked everything—including jail time—by refusing to serve in the military. He stated at the time, "I ain't got no quarrel with them Vietcong.... No Vietcong ever called me nigger."

Contrast that with today's militaristic culture in which thousands, maybe millions of young people dutifully trudge off to fight foreign wars and are lauded in the homeland, even though hardly any of them have a clue as to who or why they are fighting. As Mark Twain famously put it: "God created war so that Americans would learn geography."

Ali's act was that of a free man who trusted his own instinct and judgment, who was able and willing to think and act for himself, no matter the consequences. Today, people seem to think and act solely on the basis of which job has the best benefits and retirement package. But, for me, raising healthy children means following Ali's example and not the example set by the dominant culture—whether it's soldiers going off to war for reasons no one actually understands or people whose lives are dominated by their social standing on Facebook and Twitter. People who have come to understand and trust themselves—through years of direct, personal experience—resist groupthink, are hard to control and harder to manage, are creators and not consumers; they stand up for justice and genuinely care about the world. The question is how to raise such people. It starts with learning to trust, mostly yourself.

CHAPTER THREE

Rhythm

About fifteen years ago, I went to a weekend workshop given by the head "teacher" of an innovative pre-school in Denmark that sharpened my resolve and clarified my thinking about how to raise healthy children. Nokken, located on a roughly quarter-acre plot in Copenhagen, has developed a way of working with small children that was inspiring for me, as it was the clearest example of how the ideas I had been working with and talking about for years could be put into action. While not everyone can send their children to Nokken, or even to a school modeled on Nokken, the point is that the principles Nokken has put into practice can be used by everyone. Keeping children at home, whenever possible, is best. But the principles that guide the Nokken "school" can help us whether in the home or in an institutional setting. They are the fundamentals of raising healthy children in a world gone mad.

Nokken takes care of children from the age of one until the time they are ready to go to first grade, usually around seven. The setting is a small group of houses and outbuildings with small wooded areas and gardens. They have a small hen house, vegetable gardens, fruit trees, and a large oak tree in the central grassy courtyard. It is deliberately constructed to contain as many nooks and crannies, secret places, and separate spaces as possible. All the children, regardless of age, arrive early in the morning, generally as their parents are heading off to work. The children are greeted by one of the staff members of the school and form a small circle to greet each other and the day. After this, the children head outside to play while the adults head off to do the various work activities that make up life on a small homestead. The first important point to notice is that no matter the age of the child, even as young as one year, the adults do not automatically help the children with their outside clothes or boots. The children are encouraged (not in a verbal way) to get their own things on; they each have their own cubby with their belongings, and if they need help, they are free to ask anyone of their choosing. In the overwhelming majority of cases, one of the older children takes care of helping the younger children get ready to go outside. Without being told, they realize that some of the younger children need help, and they are willing and able to pitch in.

This is clearly a fairly minor point, and not one that all situations can replicate, but the principle behind this is that children, almost no matter their age, are encouraged to be as self-sufficient and capable as possible. When it's clear that no one will automatically put your clothes on for you, your only choice is to figure it out for yourself. If this is not possible, then asking a peer is always preferable to asking an adult. You can check this out for yourself, but young children will almost never fight with an older child to get their boots on. With an adult, they do this all the time. I will speculate about the reason in more detail later, but basically children instinctively rarely attempt to "teach," "school," or coerce other children. Since there is no power dynamic at play here, the younger children's response seems to be innately: "Might as well cooperate, as I want to go play anyways." The whole experience of getting the children ready to go outside therefore happens seamlessly, with no drama and with no input from any of the staff. Everyone just goes outside to play, no matter the weather.

The children then go off to the various parts of the property. There are no toys, but there are tools with which to do the normal work of the day. The adults do not go out to supervise the children, and other than having safety-based boundaries for the property, the children are free to do as they please, with whomever they please. The adults have work to do. They tend the garden, feed the animals, bake bread, make applesauce, mend clothes, sew, and all the other things that are needed to manage a small homestead and prepare food, clothing, and shelter for the people and animals who live there.

The next crucial point is that all the children, no matter their age, are free to join in the work of the homestead in whatever way they see fit. Some children will peel apples, others tend the garden, some like hanging out with the chickens, while others prefer to form themselves into small groups and build forts. The adults performing their daily tasks are happy to have the children join in the work. They will even at times show them how they knead bread or plant carrots, but this is done in the same way as two friends who are rock-climbing might talk together about the best toehold for this part of the rock. It's the "teaching" energy that is the key here. A number of my friend's children routinely come to help me in my Napa garden. When it comes to planting potatoes, for example, and a child comes to help (always with the caveat that they are also free to play in the mulch pile or do something else), they almost always just watch for a few minutes first. I do my best to say nothing. Then when they see how it's done, they will take the potatoes and trowel and set to work. I observe out of the corner of my eye, just to make sure they point the eyes of the potato up and plant them about the right depth. A child of five or so almost always gets it right. If they don't, I will say, "The potatoes grow from this point here, so I usually point it up, about this far down." In my experience, this is always enough. Again, like two friends talking about the best way to climb a rock face or shoot a basketball. And, again, children instinctively avoid teaching energy or language. I think they get immediately shunned and ostracized if they attempt to teach another child. To raise a healthy child, adults should learn this lesson very well.

The mornings at Nokken are spent with the children playing outside, working in the gardens, and doing other jobs that are part of the life of the homestead. No artificial jobs, no forced activities, no pressure of any sort for any child to participate in an activity that they don't feel drawn to.

A next crucial principle governing the life of this community is related to the large, central tree that dominates the grassy center of the homestead. It is a majestic tree, one with many climbing branches and often many children sitting on the different branches of the tree at one time. In one of the pictures, you could count twenty-five children sitting on various branches of the tree, seemingly just hanging out. One of the few rules at Nokken is that no one is allowed to help another child climb the tree. Even though the children love to climb the tree and it seems to be one of the favored pastimes for the children, if a child is too young, too weak, or perhaps even too timid to successfully climb even to the lowest branches, they are not to be helped. The reason for this is twofold. Firstly, and most obviously, if a child, for whatever reason, can't climb the tree, it is probably not safe for him to be up in the tree. A child who can climb to the higher branches with no help clearly has the strength and savvy to navigate the climb. A child who was either put in the tree or helped in his climb has no such confidence in himself. For this reason, it is simply not safe to help a child climb the tree. But more importantly, even though the children unsuccessfully attempt to climb the tree almost daily for six months to a year, they seem to never get tired of the quest. They circle the tree, touch the tree, maybe talk to the tree, even at times feel frustration with the tree. Yet no one helps them. They try and try. Perhaps they are simply not strong enough or observant enough yet to understand or navigate the initial ascent. Then, one day, they get it and an eruption of joy rings through the courtyard. What an accomplishment, and how wrong it would have been to help the child acquire something that was not rightfully theirs.

Last summer, while on vacation, my four-year-old, very nimble granddaughter spent a long time attempting to navigate a climbing apparatus at the park we went to daily. Finally, in a moment of stupidity on my part, I held onto her bottom, which allowed her to scale the last section of the climb. That was the last time she showed any interest in that activity. By "helping" her, I robbed her of the joy of her innate learning, her getting to know her strengths and limitations. She made me pay for this transgression by being "bored" for a few minutes and asking me what she should do. I deserved my punishment and vowed to myself never to make this stupid mistake again.

Around mid-morning, the children at Nokken gather together inside the main building, with the older children in one room and the younger children, who still benefit from taking a nap, in another room. One of the teachers sings with the children, tells them a story (as opposed to reading them a story), and they may talk or tell stories together. Each of the young children has their own mat and space, and they sleep for about half an hour. The older children return outside to play or help with the work of the homestead until lunch. The important points here are that when one uses predictability and rhythm, the flow of the day becomes much simpler. When singing, story, nap all happen in a rhythmical, predictable sequence, most children relax into this rhythm, knowing their world feels like a safe and familiar place. If there is a child who resists, I would take this as a sign that their nap is no longer needed and they can play in a different part of the house. The key is the energy or consciousness of the adults. If they are confident in their sense of the flow of the day and carry it out with no coercion, children almost always happily follow along. The key is the coercion. If there is coercion, the children rebel against this, not against taking a nap. This is a theme we will be continually exploring in the course of this book.

The other key point is that there are ways of communicating with children that will prove to be most satisfying, effective, and productive. Telling stories out of your own experience, singing your own songs is compelling for most children. This is one of the attractions of story-telling grandparents, who are much more likely than the children's parents to tell stories of their lives.

This is a lost art and one that children in general seem to crave. Every parent and adult who interacts with children should attempt to cultivate the art of telling stories, singing songs, and creating games from their own experience and childhood. Rarely can a small child resist being drawn into these tales. The next best approach is to read stories from books or sing common children's songs. Both are fine, but children, like all people, find it most rewarding to interact with other fully engaged people. If you are telling your own story from your own life, you will be engaged—less so reading from a book. And, finally, playing songs on a device or having the children listen to recorded stories will rarely capture their attention. This will typically set you up for a discipline battle, which you will inevitably lose. This is best avoided.

The rest of the day is spent outside and preparing for and eating lunch. Again, the children are free to help with the meal preparation, setting the table, sweeping the floor, and whatever else is needed to make a successful meal. Most children love food, love working with food, love having family or friends to eat with. It again all depends on the way this is presented. Children will naturally gravitate to bread-making with a baker who loves his work and is warm and inviting to the children as helpers. Opening store-bought loaves of bread is far less interesting for the child. Children want to make things; they want to be exposed to creators and makers who shape the world from their own hands. This is the quintessential human experience and one that seems to be basic nourishment for the child.

Tragically, we are becoming a society of people who create and fashion almost nothing from our own two hands and out of our own creativity. To raise healthy children, simple skills—often starting with food production—need to be re-introduced into the world of the child. Not only will you be rewarded with more nutritious food, but your child's level of engagement and satisfaction in their world will explode. Children learn through exposure and non-coerced experience on their own terms and in their own time. This is ultimately the lesson that is taught at Nokken. Expose the child to nature and a world in which things get done—not because someone decrees that now it is gardening time or now we will learn about chickens, but rather because there are tasks to be done in the garden that ultimately give us carrots to eat, because if the chickens are not fed in this rhythm, they will get sickly or die. Children, like all people, understand this, appreciate it, and want to participate in activities that from their own perspective need to get done. It's called real life.

It is the ultimate guide that helps us raise healthy children.

CHAPTER FOUR

Perseverance

In the end, it keeps coming back to the question of what we mean by a "healthy" child. Because this is such an elusive question, it might be better to start with a few qualities that at least most of us can agree on. We want our children to be strong, resilient, independent, and determined. It would be the rare parent or pedagogue who would claim the goal of his parenting or educational program is to help the child to become weak, susceptible to whatever illness comes along, to be someone who merely toes the line and is not even particularly determined to be "normal." In my field of medicine, it is very clear how to build strength and resistance in an organism. It works the same for single-celled organisms, elephants, and human beings. We learn and grow through challenges and stressors. Not the chronic, debilitating kind that are man-made and characterize our toxic cultures, but the stressors that nature puts in our path to aid in our growth.

Nowhere is the principle of developing strength through perseverance seen more clearly than in the realm of health and medicine. Unfortunately for the population, the current medical system has completely misinterpreted the meaning of the various symptoms and experiences that our bodies exhibit and this is particularly the case with children.

Conventional medicine groups various symptoms into disease categories and claim that these diseases are specific, distinct entities often caused by a specific microbe. This is commonly referred to as the germ theory. In reality, it should be referred to as the disproved germ hypothesis.

A simple example will demonstrate the error of this way of thinking. Imagine you get a splinter in your finger and for some reason don't remove it. All of us have had the experience that in due time pus will form around the splinter and will pop the splinter out thereby resolving the "illness." Clearly, the splinter is the illness and the pus is the therapy for the splinter. In contrast, we are taught in medical school that the person has an infection, caused by a bacterium, which needs to be treated with drainage and often antibiotics. It is easy to see that the bacteria are not the cause of the trouble and stopping the pus (without the drainage) would only leave the splinter in place and prolong the illness. The likelihood is that the body would make repeated attempts to expel the splinter with pus, in other words this would become a chronic illness.

The same dynamics are at work with so-called pneumonia. The person or child breathes in toxic dust, particulate matter, smoke or other debris. These are the splinters. The body in its wisdom attempts to remove these poisons and impediments and it does so in the only strategy it has, which is to make mucus, produce increased warmth to liquefy the secretions (a fever), and cough out the debris. Again, the doctors completely misinterpret what is happening; they confuse the illness (the debris) with the therapy (the so-called pneumonia or bronchitis), leading them to use antibiotics and cough suppressant drugs that thwart the body's healing attempt and prolong the illness. What should have been a simple cleansing process then becomes chronic asthma or repeated bouts of bronchitis in children.

The principle here is simple: *all* of our symptoms are the body's attempt to heal given the hand it's been dealt. If you ingest toxic food or supplements and don't move properly your body will develop deposits in the various tissues, including the joints. Then your body will create an inflammatory reaction in the tissue or joints to dissolve the deposits. This is erroneously called a disease, "arthritis" by doctors, when in reality it is just a healing strategy. All of the so-called childhood diseases are not specific entities caused by this or that virus. In fact, viruses are an imaginary construct that do not exist in the real world. These "diseases" are just common healing patterns that children use to grow, detoxify, cleanse their bodies and remove psychological, emotional, and physical impediments.

A child who never gets acutely sick, never has a fever, cough, runny nose, never has flu-like symptoms will become a weak, chronically sick person in many cases. When our children go through fevers, chickenpox, measles, etc., they get stronger, their detoxification pathways get exercised, and research has shown that these children end up with less susceptibility to all the chronic diseases from which many of the adults in our society suffer. This principle has been recognized in medicine for thousands of years and was the foundation of all medical systems until our current allopathic model. The old mantra, "Give me a medicine to produce a fever, and I can cure any disease," should be the guiding principle if our goal is to build strength, resistance, and resilience in our children. This should be the fundamental principle of pediatric health care.

About two decades ago, Dr. Larry Dossey began his tenure as the editor of the primary journal for alternative medicine in the U.S. called *Alternative Therapies*. In each issue, he wrote an editorial having to do with some interesting subject in medicine. One that caught my attention and that speaks directly to the issue of building strength, resilience, and resistance in our children was a piece he wrote entitled "Weather Deficiency Syndrome." In this piece, he discussed the experiments that had been done in the southwest desert regions of the U.S., where scientists built weather domes and raised various communities of plants, insects, animals, and people in these weather-controlled domes. The temperature was always maintained at a comfortable seventy degrees; the humidity was constant; there was no wind, no rain, no changes in the weather inside the dome at all. To their surprise, what they found was that while they did obtain rapid growth of all the plants and animals in the experiment, not only were they routinely weak and susceptible to all sorts of common illnesses, but the food plants grown in these conditions had significantly less protective nutrients in all categories as opposed to normally grown food plants. The root systems of the trees were shallow and weak; the phytochemicals and anthocyanins that plants produce to ward off disease were either absent or made in reduced quantities. The conclusion was that, even though this plant may resemble a carrot in appearance, it has little or none of the nutrients and properties that make us value carrots as a source of nourishing food.

The researchers at these weather-controlled domes also found that plants and animals grown in this fashion, without the usual exposure to the microbial world that normal plants and animals encounter, are extraordinarily susceptible to "infectious disease," and this resulted in epidemics of "infectious disease" that were more widespread and severe than usual. In other words, the strategy of having plants, animals, or humans grow up in sterile, microorganism-free environments lessens the organism's ability to resist disease. The goal of raising disease-free children, vaccinated against all possible "infectious diseases," becomes the dystopian world in which even the common cold can become a deadly enemy. This is the world that many parents and their unsuspecting pediatricians are creating for our children. It is a world that will have the inexorable and fast-approaching consequence of leaving these same children weak, vulnerable, and, above all, fearful. Fearful because of their underlying sense that they have been cheated out of the very experiences that would make them strong and resistant for their journey through life. I can hardly think of a worse fate to impose upon one's child.

This principle of growth through strength and through challenges applies to other realms of life as well. And, again, we must distinguish between the types of stressors that create growth and perseverance and the chronic, debilitating stressors that will undermine the health and confidence of the child. This is also where the principle I discussed in the opening chapter comes in: if you want to help a child become strong, resilient, and healthy, get on their side and stay there, no matter what. A child who encounters the challenges of the world with this as his foundation will be well equipped to grow and thrive. A child with no one on his side is left adrift, and this is when all possible disastrous outcomes tend to occur.

When I think back to my own childhood, one situation I can point to that helped me develop as a human being was my encounter with Willie. While it is simplistic to isolate this example and claim it led to any particular outcome, this encounter still lives vividly in my being almost fifty years after it began. There are very few other things in my life that have occupied such a large amount of my psychic space, dream life, or thoughts as my encounter with Willie.

Going through elementary school is suburban Detroit, I was shy, reserved, rarely spoke, and didn't particularly go out of my way to be with my peers. I had a supportive family situation, but neither of my parents had any clue about how to support a child emotionally; they mostly just left me alone. The thing I loved more than anything at age twelve was basketball. I was clearly the best athlete in my grade and by a large margin the best basketball player in the local twelve-and-under league. If the final score of a game was 40 to 38, I probably scored 25 to 30 of those points. I was also the top athlete in many other sports. As a twelve-year-old boy, sports occupied a large majority of my psychic space.

Starting in seventh grade, our Jewish-only elementary schools integrated, and the middle school ratio was about 80 percent white suburban Jews and 20 percent African-American children from the local projects. Theirs was a much rougher environment, and this was the late 1960s, the height of the period of racial tension in the U.S., much of which was centered in urban areas like Detroit.

For context, during my entire middle- and high-school years, we had built-in "riot" days, just as some schools will build in snow or tornado days. During these days, the racial tension in the school was so high that the administration sent us home as they attempted to defuse whatever provoked the latest flare-up. Our classes, lunchrooms, sports teams—everything was completely segregated. I never had a single African-American child in any of my classes. There were none in the chess club, drama club, or any of the sports teams (Jewish schools didn't play football at that time). The only exception was the basketball team. Our community had a long history of support for the basketball team in high school. We were a factor in the state tournaments. Many in the community came out to watch the basketball team, and the town ran vigorous programs to expose children to basketball. It was the only place in our town where the races came together outside of conflict. I was stepping into a hornet's nest.

Sometime probably in late October of seventh grade, maybe a few weeks before the tryouts for the seventh-grade basketball team, I was walking in the hallway when a group of five or six African-American boys of my age or a little older came up to me and, in a very threatening way, said, "We hear you think you're better than Floyd" (that was Willie's nickname). There were some other things said, all very threatening, about my needing to watch what I said and that bad things happen to liars. At that time, I had heard of Willie, a boy in my class who was the undisputed basketball king of the class and even amongst the older children, but I had never met him or seen him play. I was stubborn, scared out of my mind, and pretty panicked by that encounter. I used my skills at persuasion to give a twelve-year-old's nuanced explanation that while I hadn't exactly said I was better than

Willie, I was hoping to meet him and join the team. Through a combination of fear and determination, I somehow managed to escape without getting beaten up. After all, I loved basketball, and thus far no one was better than me, and I wasn't willing to concede defeat unless I felt I had to. What I didn't appreciate at the time was that I was proposing to invade their world, a world they had dominated and used as a source of pride and prestige for years. There was an inevitable conflict brewing around this.

Basketball tryouts started a few weeks later. It quickly became clear that Willie and I were by far the two best players and that Willie was actually better than me. We joined together, competed against each other in practice, and led the middle school team to a 59 to 1 record over those next three years. During this whole period, I was the subject of verbal threats, intimidation, and physical assaults (when we lined up for school, the white children would go to the front and the black children would form themselves into a kind of sheath around us, then they would push, and I was often the main target, getting punched, kicked, spit on, etc.). I never told anyone about this. Obviously, the school administrators saw what was happening, but I don't remember them saying anything specifically to me. I just dealt with it, as we all did in that very tense period of our lives.

On the basketball team, it mostly went well, at least partly because Willie, despite being an intense competitor, was an easy-going, friendly guy. He never once threatened me in any way, never said anything or did anything that provoked any sort of fear in me. He told me that my left hand stunk and that's why I would never get anywhere, and he was right. I told him he shot his jump shot too far behind his head—also true. As time went on, we became the two main players on the high school team that became ranked in the top ten of the rugged world of Michigan high school basketball. The threats, assaults, and intimidations continued all through high school. I never told anyone, not even my parents. Willie and I continued to go after each other in practice; I never lost a shooting contest with him and he never lost when we played one on one. One time, one time only, I asked him in practice if he would come over to my house some day and we could play on the little court in my driveway. He simply said, "Can't happen."

My senior-year basketball experience went badly. We started 10 to 0. The coach thought this was his ticket to getting a more lucrative job in college basketball. Then I got hurt, Willie tore up his knee, the team fell apart, and the coach quit mid-year. The racial tension in Detroit in the early 1970s was raging, and being one of only two white kids on the team was tense at best. High school ended soon after that, and I just moved on. But the thing I dreamt about the most, at least in the following two decades, was basketball, Willie, and the lack of resolution of it all. I have never been back to a class reunion, and I had no contact with anyone from my class or that school for probably three decades. Some of my best friends during high school became Harvard law graduates, neurosurgeons, and other "successful" people. The only one whose opinion I would be interested in as to how those years were for him and what he saw in or about me would be Willie. Not Charles the neurosurgeon, not my first girlfriend Pam, not Ricky the Harvard law graduate. Only Willie, only the answer to the question: "Would you have actually wanted to come to my house that day after practice?" And, "What happened to you since then, what did you do with your life, and did I have any impact on your life?" My guess is I'll never get the chance. I don't even know if Willie is still alive. But I do know that without this intensely challenging and stressful experience, I would not be who I am today. My guess is the importance of this situation was the combination of having to face an intense and frightening challenge and the fact that Willie, in his own way, and for his own reasons, accepted me into his basketball world. Maybe it was because I could help him get a scholarship if we were a good team, but maybe it was because Willie understood more than he let on that there was a human situation here and that if he accepted me, I would be safe and that I could even grow as a player. He never wavered and I can't thank him enough.

Now, I can only ask you to imagine a world in which we never allow our children to have experiences like this. I'm not saying getting punched, intimidated, and kicked is a good thing or something we should deliberately expose our children to. But if resolve and perseverance are things we value in our children, a world without conflict and challenge will never work. If you are your child's ally, no matter what, and if you watch out for blatantly unsafe situations (clearly an issue in some of our communities), then you can help your child grow, thrive, and prosper in a way that is simply not possible in the conflict-, disease-free model that is currently being proposed.

CHAPTER FIVE

Play

Over the years, I'm sure that I've said and written a number of things that many people didn't agree with. The single thing I'd ever said or written that had drawn the most negative comments, reviews, and angry questioning (prior to the year 2020) is my line in the book *The Nourishing Traditions Book of Baby and Childcare* advising parents not to play with their children. I went on to explain that I didn't mean parents or adults shouldn't interact with their children, only that play is a sacred activity for children, one that adults seem to have lost the knack for. As a result, we adults should not interfere with, guide, or otherwise disturb the play, especially of a young child.

After more than a decade of living with this statement, and the often-negative backlash I got from it, I have decided to revise that statement and try to further refine what I now mean. My new statement is: children should not be encouraged in any way to play, at all. While I can almost hear the rising chorus of derision that this new statement will provoke, I hope you permit me to once again explain myself. Play has become almost a sacred cow in the thought of modern educators. Childhood experts, in particular those with a more progressive bent, write articles and books on the crucial importance of play to the young child. Major sports institutions, like the NFL, sponsor "play 60" campaigns that encourage all children to "get out and play" for 60 minutes per day. I can't think of anyone of any stature or relevance in the modern or "alternative" culture that doesn't encourage us to let our children play, and the more the better.

So, why would I write such a provocative statement? Maybe this is about semantics, but I have become convinced that unless we parse this out, we will never get anywhere close to our goal of raising healthy children in a toxic world. One of the elements of this toxic world is our attitude toward and understanding of play.

Any definition of play immediately points out the contrast between play and work. The dictionary definition of play (according to Siri) is "to engage in activity for enjoyment and recreation rather than for a serious or practical purpose." In contrast, the definition of work is "activity involving mental or physical effort done in order to achieve a purpose or result." Just yesterday I was in the garden doing the usual winter clean-up—weeding, planting carrots, etc. We have a small group of friends who come and help and share in our harvest. One of the families has a wonderful three-year-old boy who loves to help in the garden. He is a lively, spirited little guy who clearly knows his own mind and what he wants to do. Yesterday, he marched into the garden and grabbed a trowel and started digging around in some of the beds. The adults around him just greeted him, and engaged in friendly banter. After a while, he put down the trowel, went over to the tool bucket, grabbed a pair of huge, sharp hedge clippers and trundled off to trim some plants. I didn't mind the trimming-plants part, but it looked like he might shear off a finger or his nose, so I gently guided him away from the clippers and he ran to the wood-chip pile. After a while of loading some chips into the wheelbarrow, he joined a group of adults in digging weeds from the pathways. All the time, he carried on a lively banter with anyone around, occasionally ate the few strawberries still on the plants, and basically did this for about three hours. As far as I could tell, he had a great time and never once in those three hours did anyone have to manage him in any way, except for my hiding the clippers. I obviously can't be sure about this, but my guess is if you asked him if he spent the last three hours doing activity that had a serious or practical purpose, he would emphatically say, Yes, and, if asked, would consider the person asking the question a condescending jerk and someone he wants nothing to do with. He absolutely had a purpose to his activities, sometimes it was to pull weeds, sometimes to find yummy strawberries, sometimes to see how high he could throw bark mulch, sometimes to feel his little legs run as fast as they could. How much more of a serious or practical endeavor could one possibly want?

The problem here is that our toxic culture has created an artificial distinction between work and play that doesn't exist in reality. In fact, I would even go further and propose that the distinction between work and play arose only to serve the interests of those who want to convince the general population that they should do something called "work," to make a "living," and their reward will be the occasional time to "play" at something they actually want to do.

This thing called "work" is done mostly to get access to money, without which you can't eat or find shelter or clothing. This same money, as I have repeatedly pointed out, is given to the 1 percent of the 1 percent of people to create out of thin air (and to make available relatively freely to the other 99 percent of the 1 percent), while the general population—that is, 99 percent of the people—must "work" to obtain this money. The corollary to my statement that children should not play is: neither should adults work. As I have also pointed out in previous books, and as brilliantly depicted by Ivan Illich in his book *The Right to Useful Unemployment*, the happiness and fulfillment of the people in any given culture is directly tied to the level of employment in that culture. The higher percentage of employed people in a country, the higher the level of personal misery in the people. The "jobbed" are miserable because they hate their tedious jobs and have profound, deep resentment for being "forced" to spent the vast majority of their lives working at this job.

The unemployed are miserable because they are deemed useless and misfits for not contributing to society. This must be why politicians of all stripes continually call for more jobs and more jobs. Jobs or work is the holy grail, never mind that the only people it actually serves are the people who create the money, who use other people's labor to consolidate their power and make more money. Allowing yourself to get pulled into the work/play dynamic leads you into this trap and soon you will find yourself in a ditch with an angry and resentful child.

Instead, like my gardening friend, let all the activities that the child AND the grown-up engage in be active, meaningful, creative, self-generated pursuits that are done both for enjoyment and to achieve a purpose or result. That is how most of the human beings who have ever inhabited our world spent most of their lives—Plorking. When work is artificially divorced from play, my sense is people enjoy neither. For sure, the very privileged few get to do enjoyable work, but this is an overwhelming minority of the people in the work force. The rest, the vast majority, have this nagging feeling that this is not the way life is supposed to be. Work all day to escape debt, produce nothing, create nothing, think about things that you are told to think about and then have the privilege of going to a sporting event, or heaven forbid to "play" golf, which seems to be just another avenue for misery for most people. Every single culture that uses this model ends up consuming more and more of the earth's resources, creating more and more garbage, and becoming more and more violent. It doesn't matter if they are communists or capitalists, free marketeers or socialists, whether they want to pay people a "livable wage" or outright starve them. If people's lives are separated between work and play, you will create a consumer society that over time devours the earth and angers the children. Public education in which the central lesson is "work," and if you're good you get to go out to recess and "play," only creates more anger and resentment in children. All anyone wants to do is meaningful, creative activities, which arise out of one's own initiative. These activities are both fun AND achieve a purpose and a result. That is the normal, healthy activity that allows all humans, young and old, to thrive. Separating the two only creates misery.

This will and should bring up a whole list of questions and objections. These include: How can one practically have children plork all the time, how will we support ourselves if no one is making money, and if we only do creative, fun, purposeful things, who will clean the toilets?

And, finally, the "big objection," the thought that has ruined more lives than perhaps any other human thought: "I must discipline my children to be responsible adults, to learn to make a living, otherwise they will amount to nothing." As Sarah Palin once said (I can't believe I'm quoting Sarah Palin, last time, I promise), "How's that working out for ya?"

My first response, as I pointed out in *Human Heart, Cosmic Heart*, is that a world without money was the norm for the bulk of human existence. Mostly people lived their lives, did what they had to do to find food, love, support, shelter, clothes, and comfort, and no money was needed.

Money, which started out as a simple tool of exchange, a kind of generic placeholder representing the goods one would have normally bartered with, has evolved into a self-perpetuating, centralized, monopolistic control-mechanism that places most people "in debt" and makes them wage-slaves. At some point, this edifice will have to be torn down to create the type of world most of us would rather inhabit. For now, let's turn to the more "practical," immediate issues concerning our children. My premise is that if we expose our children to the world of nature, music, song, food, creativity (making clothes, baskets, forts, whatever), they will naturally gravitate to the things most meaningful for them. We need to be very clear that none of these activities carries any more weight or gravitas than any other. A young child who loves flowers, who plants them, cares for them, picks them, arranges them is no more or less important than another child who wants to build structures. This is just individual expression and needs to be honored. Your primary job, besides keeping the child safe (i.e., not allowing them to cut their nose off with hedge clippers), is to expose them to as many of these types of activities as you can muster. With enough diversity, it is rare to find a child who doesn't find their niche. Some children focus on one activity, some change activities and interests seemingly by the minute. As far as is practical, either way is fine.

Then let them plork; offer as little guidance (besides safety concerns) as possible, but also, just as when doing an activity with a good friend, there are times when dialogue, suggestions, demonstrations, etc. can be a wonderful step. As long as it's clear that this is your opinion or how you do it, the child will almost always show interest and appreciate the input. If a child is cutting flowers, it could be helpful to demonstrate that flowers last longer when cut at the base rather than right below the flower—most children would figure this out anyway. These activities can be "practical" things like building forts, planting gardens, or they can be painting pictures or constructing elaborate farm scenes with their wooden animals.

Some children gravitate toward wooden animals and may even want to try their hand at making them; others want to feed chickens. The point is that these are profoundly practical and serious activities, which is part of the reason, if not the main reason, they are so compelling and fun. Children love doing these types of activities; and they love making up games—another profound way human beings learn to socialize, establish boundaries and rules, and cooperate in a shared activity. This is serious business, one that all human beings should partake in as much as possible.

Like my young friend in the garden, children approached in this manner generally have tremendous attention spans, need no disciplinary intervention at all, are productive and helpful even at age three, and everyone has a great time getting to know each other's interests and quirks.

And, I will guarantee this, if your child's life is approached in this manner, with this mindset that we are going to engage in real activities that are not only needed but fun, they will be much, much more likely to help clean the toilet than the child you attempt to punish when they fail to do their chores. In fact, from everything I see with today's children, because they are approached with the mindset of the dichotomy of work and play, most children rarely do anything that could be considered useful or productive (besides school, which we will explore in great depth later on). This is a horrible and debilitating position for any human being to be in.

Children, like all people, crave to be doing fun, productive, useful, and serious activities. The money, or the "living," will come; these will be the healthy, creative people who will find a new road forward for our culture. It starts by getting rid of play (and work)!

CHAPTER SIX

Integrity

The other day I read an article in an emergency medicine journal that outlined the story behind the "clot-busting" drugs that are currently being used to treat stroke patients in emergency rooms. There are two main types of strokes. The most common, called ischemic strokes, are thought to happen because of plaque formation in the arteries leading up to the brain. As a result of the plaque-based blockages, the blood doesn't get through and a section of the brain dies as a result of poor blood supply. This can also happen as a result of small pieces of plaque breaking off of a larger clot and completely plugging one of the vessels leading to the brain. This constitutes about 60 percent of strokes. The other 40 percent are called hemorrhagic strokes, which occur as a result of the rupture of one of the blood vessels in the brain. This also leads to poor perfusion of an area of the brain, resulting in the death of those brain cells. For decades, various drug manufacturers have attempted to come up with clot-busting drugs that would quickly restore blood flow for those with ischemic strokes while not increasing the inevitable risk of bleeding that occurs when you thin the blood. Generally speaking, the trials on all such drugs showed no overall benefit to stroke patients, as the decrease of one type led to an increase of the other type.

About a decade ago, Genentech, a large biotech drug company, came out with a new clot-busting drug and produced a clinical trial that showed it had a small benefit. Subsequent studies, done by independent investigators, failed to demonstrate this same benefit. The one small study was enough to secure approval for its use from the FDA, and it quickly became the standard of care for the treatment of ischemic stroke patients in ERs across the country. This meant the drug was a multibillion-dollar seller for Genentech. The problem was that ER doctors across the country complained about its use. They saw no benefit and many of their patients had bleeding episodes as a result of the drug. There were bitter complaints and editorials demanding a new, large, independent study done to demonstrate once and for all that the drug was both safe and effective. Genentech up to this point has refused to do this study.

When asked why they wouldn't do it, here is what one of the senior scientists at Genentech had to say: "We don't know how another trial would turn out. And if we don't come out ahead, we would have a tremendously self-inflicted wound.... Another study may be a good thing for America, but it wasn't going to be a good thing for us."

In a similar vein, there is the published deposition from one of the world's foremost leaders in vaccine development. This physician has spent his entire career, spanning over five decades, creating, developing, promoting, and doing studies on vaccines. He is by all accounts the dean of vaccine research in the world at this time. The setting was a deposition, under oath, where he served as an expert witness in a dispute between two estranged parents. The father wanted their children vaccinated; the mother didn't. The questioning was conducted by a lawyer for the mother, who was clearly well versed in the vaccine literature. As part of the questioning, the lawyer delved into this doctor's history of vaccine research. Under oath, this respected physician admitted to doing multiple vaccine trials in the early part of his career on handicapped, disabled children, and "mentally retarded" children. He also was the lead investigator on studies done on children in remote areas of Africa, and other less "civilized" places. These were early trials of the vaccines, meaning they were done to assess the safety of the vaccines. Some apparently passed the trials and were found to be "safe," others not. The lawyer produced statements from the doctor attesting to the ethics of these trials based on his view that these children would never be fully functioning members of our society and therefore medical experimentation on them—and, in the case of the African children, without their parents' full knowledge or consent—was warranted for the greater good. To be fair, the physician has since had what he describes as an epiphany and would no longer conduct safety trials on African children or disabled children. He does, however, grow his "viral" cultures on fetal tissue, including the heart, brain, tongue, and other organs of the aborted, harvested fetuses. He has no ethical qualms about this, nor any safety concerns, even though he admits that this inevitably means that human tissue from these aborted fetuses will show up in the final vaccine and the consequences of this for the recipient are at this time unknown.

And, finally, the well-known case of the medicine Vioxx, made by Merck, the world's largest manufacturer of vaccines, tells a similar story. In the investigation into the over 50,000 deaths that were directly caused by the use of Vioxx for various pain syndromes, internal emails from Merck executives told a clear story about their knowledge of and conclusions about the link between their medicine and fatal heart attacks. These emails show beyond a shadow of a doubt that even before releasing this drug, they had sufficient evidence to know of the harm it would cause.

They understood that there would eventually be a time when they would be required to compensate victims and to pay fines as a result of concealing evidence of the known harm of their drug. They knew there would be thousands of victims—heartbreak and loss incurred by countless families. But they calculated that the return from the sale of the drug compared to the total cost to produce, research, market, and distribute the drug, even with the projected fines and settlements, would result in billions of dollars of profit, and this would be an overall win for the company. Clearly, they were right: it is estimated that Vioxx made Merck over five billion dollars after all these expenses.

Now, compare these three scenarios with the simple statement and story of Mohammed Ali in chapter two. The reason I bring this up in a book on raising healthy children is that I have asked many parents: How would you feel if you received a letter documenting how your child prevented the truth from coming out about the dangers of a drug used to treat vulnerable stroke patients? Or that your child grew up to do medical experimentation on poor, "retarded," or disabled children? Or how would you feel knowing your child grew up to be the accountant who ran the numbers for Merck and decided that Vioxx should be a "go"? Without exception, the response I have gotten is: "I would be horrified." That's the point. If we don't want to raise children to do horrifying things at some point, somebody is going to have to try to understand how and why this keeps happening. I used medical examples because that's the field I'm most knowledgeable in. I'm sure that no matter which area of our culture we examine, similar horrifying stories would surface. The question is how to raise children who have integrity, how to raise Mohammed Ali's and not researchers who test vaccines on unsuspecting children.

Of course, I have no simple answer for this question, nor do I claim any special relationship to integrity myself. Furthermore, like most questions about how to produce certain outcomes in individual people, there are personal *and* societal factors that drive these outcomes. We live in a culture whose fundamental ethos is: You are in a cutthroat competition called life, and it behooves you to do whatever you can to succeed. For many, if not most people, there are very few effective social support systems, family support systems, or any other avenues for getting one's needs met besides one's own wit and will.

This will inevitably produce "successful" people who do monstrous things. My guess is the Genentech doctor, the vaccine developer, and the Merck executives are all considered very successful people with good families, status in their communities, perhaps even examples of warmth and generosity due to their philanthropy. None of this allows us to escape the conclusion that in a just world, a world populated by healthy people, these people are all in need of restorative justice, a process in which they are removed from normal society, and every one of their "victims" would have the opportunity to explain to them, face to face, just exactly what the result of their actions has been on their families. These people would not be "freed" until each and every "victim" agrees that they now understand fully the consequences of their choices. Just imagine our world if this was the process we had to undergo in the event of lapses in our integrity. Imagine a world that really takes seriously the principle that needlessly doing harm or violence to any other being is itself grounds for the need to participate in a restorative justice procedure. But, given that the world of justice and non-violence is not going to emerge anytime soon, are there things we can do to foster integrity in our children?

I would propose that the experience of shame, and its cousin humiliation, is perhaps the root cause of the development of adults who are willing to inflict violence and suffering on others. This entire book, everything from the exploration of diet, vaccines, how to treat children with fevers, rhythm, plork, etc. is all geared toward raising healthy children who do not turn out to do horrifying things. But, specifically, to raise a child with integrity means to avoid any use of either shame or humiliation in your interaction with your child or with anyone else in your life.

Similar to making the commitment to being on your child's side no matter what, modeling integrity means modeling, speaking, living a life that puts no one down, no matter what. This is not the same as being wishy-washy. This means expressing vehement objection to actions or words spoken by another, including one's child. In every case, this should be done as clearly and factually as possible, with no sense of shame, humiliation, or belittlement. One has to consciously cultivate this approach to life, and the more deeply one feels the injustices, the harder this is. The child, though, must get the message loud and clear that while in our family we are free to discuss all issues, we avoid personal attacks, personal shaming or humiliation, whether it's directed toward our fiercest enemies or our closest loved ones. In this sphere, paradoxically, it's often those closest to us that we tend to shame and humiliate the most. The words, "You should be ashamed of yourself," words I clearly remember hearing as a child, should be stricken from the vocabulary of all those who even get near a child. Shaming, in words or actions, is the opposite of being on your child's side. Never use these words. Instead, talk intensely about the events, actions, and motivations in our lives. Explore as deeply as you can how we decide one course of action over another; never question the motives or the integrity of your child. They will reward you with a lifetime of actions motivated by deep deliberation on the right action and how that is accomplished.

Finally, I have two other quick suggestions that I trust will foster integrity in our children. The first is to let them hear stories of men, women, and children who took actions out of a deep sense of integrity. The only caveat is, as much as possible, make sure there is no ambiguity in the "cause" being fought for. Ali's cause was fairness and justice; a soldier fighting for freedom in Syria may turn out to be a pawn in a scenario he has no awareness of. One of the best stories, appropriate for any child over the age of six, is *To Kill a Mockingbird*. Real stories of integrity stick with us for life and create the possibility that one day, faced with the inevitable hard decision, a decision that pits them against the common mores of their society, your child may look inward and ask themselves, "What would Atticus Finch do in this situation?"

The other suggestion—again, one that we all need to cultivate almost daily—is to show real interest in your child when greeting them after a significant absence. This includes when your child wakes up in the morning and when they come home from prolonged activity or from a trip. Smile. If appropriate, give them a hug; take a moment to make it very clear that they are important in your life and that you are glad they are with you. Over time, this produces the same sense in the child that I am so keen on developing in this book: "My Dad is on my side; we are doing this journey called life together; from that place, I can be a force for good in this world."

CHAPTER SEVEN

Food Fights

Ever since my son Joe finally showed me, when he was about ten years old, the cause and treatment for food fights, I have had almost a 100 percent cure rate for stopping food fights in the families I've worked with. Before this epiphany, I, like many people, had seen our family dinners degenerate into unhappy battles based on my attempts to get my children to eat the food I "knew" was good for them and their refusal to cooperate. I have seen many families over the years who have become so beaten down by this dynamic that they resort to feeding their children only macaroni and cheese, just to avoid these nightly battles. I have seen many parents confronting chronic illness in their children, desperately wanting to change the diet of the child but finding that the child simply won't cooperate with the suggested dietary changes. In probably one quarter of the children who have been brought to me over the years for help with their chronic illness, the primary underlying issue was their refusal to eat the "good" food served by their parents. This problem is reinforced when one looks at surveys of what American children currently eat. A high percentage of the food consumed by today's children are high sugar foods with little or no nutritional value. Overall, we are as far away as we could be from the nutrient-dense, whole-food, locally grown diet of our healthy ancestors. There are many reasons for this, but foremost among them is whenever new diets or foods are introduced, the children balk, food fights ensue, and the parents give in. The solution to this problem can't be just to give more lectures about good food and traditional diets—to a large extent, most of my parents already know this. The problem is the food fights. This must be confronted head on.

The entire solution to the problem of food fights lies in understanding that food fights are almost never about food. Rather, as Marshall Rosenberg correctly pointed out, food fights are about autonomy. Food fights are about the right of every human being, including a human being aged three, seven, or fourteen, to decide for themselves what to eat, with no outside interference. This right, which seems to be tied to an innate learning process that allows the young person to learn about the relationship between what they eat and how they feel, is so crucial that some children will practically starve themselves to obtain this right. Once one recognizes that this is the underlying dynamic behind food fights, the solution becomes simple and obvious. With Joe, I simply admitted he was correct and from that point on, I would not engage in any sort of attempt to force him to eat anything. This included completely eliminating any sort of punishment or reward (more on this general subject later) from his food choices. This meant no "go to your room if you don't eat your carrots," no "you can have desert if you eat broccoli," no positive comments such as "good job eating those beets," no "we can go to the ball game if you eat your meat." For a young child, I wouldn't verbally state your commitment to eliminate any coercion around food; just do it. For an older child, you may want to casually state it once. It's likely your child won't believe you anyway, at which point you just make it a practice and they will see if you really learned your lesson.

Soon after I told Joe, once, that I was no longer going to coerce him to eat anything, he said at dinner, "Are you going to make me eat my broccoli?"

"How would I do that?" I said.

He laughed because obviously it's absurd to imagine me stuffing broccoli down his throat with a potato masher or something. "Well, can I go outside if I don't eat all my dinner?"

"I think so," I replied. "I guess it depends whether you want to go outside after dinner."

"Are you going to be upset if I don't eat my food?"

"No, it's your choice from now on."

These types of conversations went on for about a week. He mostly probed to see how committed I was to this practice of non-interference with his food consumption. I stuck to my commitment. The immediate objection I hear from parents is: How can you possibly think that it is reasonable to allow a young child to decide on their food consumption? The answer is, as they generally have already discovered: you have no choice in the matter. Almost all children are more committed to their freedom than you are to good food. Whatever other strategy you use, if it's about food, you will lose. However, if it is clear to your child, at any age, that you not only have heard their plea for autonomy, but you agree with it and even celebrate it, then this problem will resolve itself. What could be more wonderful than a child deciding to stand up for their own freedom?!

And here, then, is the key: once your child is convinced the battle for autonomy is over, they will eat whatever you give them. After a week or so, Joe would say things like, "You know, Dad, I like kale more than chard," or "I like chicken more than beef," etc. I took these requests seriously. We talked about the fact that kale and chard are similar from a plant or nutritional perspective, and I was happy to give him kale instead of chard, and I told him to let me know if he ever wanted to go back to chard. The point is that most children frankly could care less about these kinds of details, and they don't want to be bothered with them. Food quality is your role. They don't know what food is supposed to be good and what food isn't, and mostly they don't care. Children just don't want to have their autonomy taken from them. Once you give this gift to them, they give you back the decision about what food to eat in the home, which they never wanted in the first place.

In the beginning of this process, most parents will have to take the uncomfortable step of presenting their child with food for dinner and the child refusing to eat it. At that point, inwardly and outwardly, you have to be totally at peace with this choice. That doesn't mean you have to give them something else to eat. After all, you planned and executed a perfectly good dinner (hopefully), with lots of delicious fats, many flavors and food groups. You have no need to make something different. This can be quickly and easily explained. At that point, their choice is to eat or not, with no hint of any consequences at all (except maybe their own natural feeling of hunger). This is the hard part, the inward stance that this is all good—I did my part, and my child is doing their part. In my experience, this may result in a hungry child one night, but almost never for more than two days. Once they trust that you got the message, it's simply time to eat and move on.

One could ask how I am so confident this will work? Besides the fact that it worked with Joe and scores of patients for the last two decades, I also lived in Swaziland for two years in a mud hut. Our homestead was one of a traditional extended Swazi family, and we ate most of our meals together for these two years. The Swazis, like many traditional societies, have lots of extended family members living in one homestead. There were always between two and five children of various ages living with us at any given time. The children ranged in age from one to eighteen. There were grandparents, uncles, cousins, aunts, and friends all mixed in together, especially at the evening meal. This was not a wealthy family by any means. They grew their own food, which consisted of corn meal, beans, and a variety of greens and root vegetables they collected from their fields.

They ate meat when they could get it and raised pigs and chickens for meat and eggs. I must admit, the meals were pretty much the same night after night, and pretty boring. I never once saw, in my two years and probably hundreds of dinners, a child complain about or not eat their food. As my understanding of Siswati (their language) was far from perfect, it's possible there was a complaint at some point, but not that I was aware of. I can imagine that if a child had said, "I don't like porridge or slimy greens," within seconds someone would have whisked away their plate and eaten it themselves. If this child had said, "I want millet porridge instead of corn porridge" (especially in a whiny tone), there would have been uproarious laughter around the fire. Not exactly laughing at the child, but more just the creativity and outrageousness of the request. As far as the grandmother cooking millet porridge, not a chance. The children learn quickly that we are grateful for our food, even the slimy greens. Without these, life may not go so well, so why not eat it; it's just food.

I realize we are not Swazis, and we are able to give our children almost any food they want. Don't do it. Choose what you think is the right diet for them. Take all aspects of food into account—your access to local produce, what you are able to grow yourself, environmental issues, your family budget, your cooking expertise and style—and devise the most nutritious, economical, flavorful diet you can. Your days of debilitating food fights will soon be over.

As a side note to this, Joe is now the head of recipe development and food production at our family business, Dr. Cowan's Garden. He recently opened a bakery that provides traditionally made unleavened bread made from heirloom, mostly biodynamic grains. A few years ago, he came home for Thanksgiving and from scratch cooked the entire meal for us and a few friends. He is an accomplished, self-trained chef. Maybe that was why the food battles were so meaningful to him at that young age. He needed me on his side so he could start the process of really learning about food.

CHAPTER EIGHT

Punishments and Rewards

"We destroy the disinterested (I do not mean uninterested) love of learning in children, which is so strong when they are small, by encouraging and compelling them to work for petty and contemptible rewards—gold stars, or papers marked 100 and tacked to the wall, or A's on report cards...in short, for the ignoble satisfaction of feeling that they are better than someone else.... We kill not only their curiosity but their feeling that it is a good and admirable thing to be curious, so that by the age of ten, most of them will not ask questions and will show a good deal of scorn for the few who do."
—John Holt, *How Children Fail*

"Reward-and-punishment is the lowest form of education."
—Chuang Tzu

Imagine how you would feel if somewhere between ten and one hundred times per day, every day, your colleagues, boss, supervisor, or manager said "good job" to you for doing something that was part of your normal, routine activities. Even worse, imagine that instead of hearing "good job," you were given gold stars, ribbons, or some other trivial "reward" again for doing tasks that are part of your daily routine. Imagine that these comments or rewards were given openly in front of all your colleagues and that you received either way more or way less of these comments and rewards than your coworkers. My guess is most of my readers would, if possible, soon be looking for a different line of work, or at least a different place to work.

Now imagine that in this same work place, if you were either slow in performing your tasks, late in finishing your tasks, didn't understand fully the nature of your task—and there was no one available to explain the task—or simply thought it was a stupid task to begin with, this same colleague, boss, supervisor, or manager, in front of all your friends and colleagues, admonished you publicly and sent you to the break-room closet for ten minutes to "think about your behavior." How about if implicit in this admonition was the threat that if you didn't start performing this task better, the colleague, boss, supervisor, or manager was going to make you stay after work to do the task over and over until they were satisfied that this would never happen again. Have you quit yet?

How about if you were told that if you continued failing to perform this task, you would either be starved, deprived of access to your favorite activities, or, horror of horrors, be forced to repeat this same task the following year because if you didn't learn to succeed at performing this task, you would never amount to anything. Remember, you either didn't understand the task or, more likely, thought it was a stupid task in the first place. If you haven't quit yet, then my guess is that it's only because you have deemed the consequences of being "unjobbed" so horrific that you are willing to put up with almost anything.

The amazing thing is that this is what the normal child living in the "civilized" US puts up with almost every day of their lives. Frankly, I'm always amazed we don't have more violent episodes involving children in our society. How does anyone put up with this?

Now, of course, modern educators, and many parents, will argue that unless we teach discipline to our children and force them to learn how to become productive citizens, they will never amount to anything. As Marshall Rosenberg often said, the most evil is often done by the nicest people, often with the best intentions. These educators and childhood experts will demand evidence showing that children can in fact grow up free of punishment and reward without becoming psychopaths. For those interested, I would refer you to the book *Punished by Rewards* by Alfie Kohn, if you want documentation of the gross harm done to children who are raised with the punishment-and-reward philosophy.

Contrast this approach to life with the current strategy of sending recalcitrant children off to the "slow" class, to be labeled and treated as a "stupid" person until they learn to toe the line.

Or this statement by Anne Sullivan, the legendary teacher of Helen Keller:

> I am beginning to suspect all elaborate and special systems of education. They seem to me to be built upon the supposition that every child is a kind of idiot who must be taught to think. Whereas, if the child is left to himself, he will think more and better, if less showily. Let him go and come freely, let him touch real things and combine his impressions for himself, instead of sitting indoors at a little round table, while a sweet-voiced teacher suggests that he build a stone wall with his wooden blocks or make a rainbow out of strips of colored paper, or plant straw trees in bead flower pots. Such teaching fills the mind with artificial associations that must be got

rid of, before the child can develop independent ideas out of actual experience.

Many modern parents and educators, exactly as Anne Sullivan suggests, seem to think that the children in their lives are some type of idiot who must be educated to enlightenment. It is difficult to fathom just how much harm this fundamental concept has done to children and people. To raise a healthy child in a toxic world, it is crucial that we see this in a new way.

Over my many years of practice, I have seen hundreds, maybe by now a thousand children as new patients. My estimate is that in well over half of the first visits of children above the age of three, the parents admonish, correct, threaten, or reward their child an average of ten to twenty times in the space of the hour appointment. I once, for fun, counted the number of times each parent in one month said "no" to their children in this first visit. The average was about fifteen per hour. The amazing thing is as far as I could tell, not once did the child ever obey or even acknowledge the admonition. "Johnny, don't touch the doctor's tools," "put down that stethoscope," "stop playing with those tongue depressors." Never mind the fact that I know full well that children are very interested in these things and I leave out my old tools just so they can mess around with them while in my office. Sometimes, I'll even say something like, "I put the stethoscope in my ears like this so I can hear better." It never seems to matter; the parents intervene anyway.

Sometimes I hear the parents promise to get the child a treat or ice cream, or to go to the park if they are "good" during the exam. It never works. The child almost always goes right on as if it were a fly buzzing in their ear. I have often wondered why parents and educators persist in using strategies like punishments and rewards in spite of their obvious failures. My guess, having done so myself as a parent, is that we parents are scared to death that our child will somehow turn out to be an embarrassment to us, which will unmask us as incompetent parents.

Either it's that or it's the belief that if we somehow don't teach our children to be normal, civilized people, they will turn out to be the savages toward which they are naturally inclined. Ironically, both of these concepts turn out to be self-defeating: the first results in a feeling of shame and inadequacy on the part of the parent, leading to paralysis; the second is a martial, punitive view of the world, which inexorably produces people who punish and destroy others. There is nothing more absurd than physically, verbally, or emotionally punishing children so as to prevent them from growing up to be physically, verbally, or emotionally abusive to others. American culture, if nothing else, is a dramatic example of how this mindset clearly doesn't work and only results in a violent, warlike, abusive way of life. That is not what I mean by healthy children.

The question, though, is whether there is an alternative model for "raising" children, especially with regard to dealing with behaviors that we would rather not see. This becomes the crucial question. To be clear, in this next section in which I give suggestions for an alternative way to approach "discipline," I am leaning on four types of experience: the first is my experience as a parent and grandparent; the second is my observations as a doctor over the course of more than thirty-five years; the third is my experience as an observer of Waldorf schools; and the last is my understanding of my fellow human beings gained over sixty-three years of life. My first and probably most important reflection on this issue is that I see no reason to treat your or any child any different, in the vast majority of situations, than you would treat a trusted friend. You would never tell a friend to go to their room if they talked too loudly, so why is this OK with your child? Most people rarely if ever admonish their friends or use rewards to get them to do things. Rarely with a friend do you say "no."

This is my first suggestion, one I followed myself about twenty-five years ago when I decided to rarely if ever say "no." As a transition phase, I often tell the parents of my young patients: For the first month, you are allowed to say "no" once a day. After that, once a week for another month, then not at all. To get even more specific, if one of your children is actually doing bodily harm to another child, it is perfectly reasonable to separate them with the use of the least force possible.

The use of this type of force in the nonviolent communication world is called "the protective use of force." It means if someone is going to harm you or your child, it is clear that you must use whatever force is necessary to prevent this harm from being done. If one sees this clearly, protective use of force prevents violence being done to your child *and* it protects the perpetrator from doing violence, which is harmful for them as well. It should be very clear, however, that with most children, this type of situation is rare, but also that, if it arises, you must act swiftly and with purpose.

The more common situations that evoke some form of discipline are far from potentially violent or catastrophic occurrences. Here, the protective use of force is not appropriate. For all these situations, the first thing to do is take a step back before you intervene in any way. Save your one "no" for when it is absolutely needed, if at all, and I can guarantee that it will carry more weight and be much more effective than a "no" used fifty or a hundred times per day. If your two boys are wrestling in the living room, with no real chance of danger, is it really necessary for you to intervene and stop this behavior? Even if you try, are you actually effective by saying "no" (in all its various forms) anyway? My observation is that the children simply ignore you or actually accentuate their activities just to get your goat. Take the possibility of getting your goat out of the equation, and that alone will stop most of the things you are objecting to.

The observation that has convinced me of the truth of this approach was gained through observation of at least fifty different Waldorf teachers. Two of them—one being my wife Lynda, the other a very experienced teacher in New Hampshire—as far as I could see never disciplined their students or said any form of "no." They both told me that when the children were very young, they did very occasionally use some form of disciplinary activity, but within a short time, this simply never came up again. I have asked myself for years how they did this; neither could give me particularly clear answers. My observation told me that they had a way of making the classes so engaging that it probably never occurred to the children to "misbehave." It was simply too much fun to stand on their desks and learn to dance the Hula for them to bother to "misbehave." They also spoke about having high expectations for the children in their classes.

Inwardly, they saw all their children as being gifted in some way, able to contribute positively to the social whole of the class, and somehow the children acted in this manner.

Interestingly, they were the only two teachers who never sent a child to the doctor to get help fixing their "bad behavior." They just kind of shrugged and said they couldn't think of any particular child who needed this type of intervention.

In contrast, I saw teachers who every minute or so were scolding, admonishing, threatening, or proposing rewards to their students. They usually ended up quitting teaching fairly soon, as it was clear it was not rewarding for them or their students. These classes were chaotic with all kinds of weird stuff happening. Inevitably, these teachers sent many children to the doctor to "get fixed." We all know people who have a way with children, people whom children just seem to love to be around. Watch them; they almost always have no need for punishment or reward.

Rather, they enjoy the activities; they share them with interested children, which means almost all of the children; they laugh, cry, sing, tell stories, and treat each other as you would treat a valued friend. I understand we can't all be these people, but we can learn from them and attempt to follow their lead. We can also be aware that this ability is largely an inner quality, and this, too, must be cultivated. It's hard to be a grown-up; it's hard to be a parent; it can even be hard to be a friend. That doesn't mean we are not all called to try.

I have a few recent stories from my life that hopefully will demonstrate another approach to dealing with young children when they inevitably do things that are difficult for us adults to accept. I offer these in the spirit of possibility and not with the claim that somehow I have it all figured out. In fact, nothing could be further from the truth, as I didn't seem to have much natural talent for interacting with young children. I, like many of us, went through years of exasperation and confusion as I tried to come to some understanding of how to live in a harmonious and productive manner with my young children. I am offering these stories in the spirit of "if I can learn a better way, then anyone can."

The first story is about an experience with my grandson Ben. At the time, he was around four and was staying with us, along with his brother and my daughter, due to their family circumstances.

Most every morning, I would go get Ben from the cottage where he slept early in the morning as we were the two earliest risers. Mostly, we would come to our house and be downstairs with his blocks and wooden animals, building the farm for the day. Sometimes he would use his crayons to draw pictures. One morning, I heard a "Grandpa" in an unusual voice, and I knew I should go look. Ben was standing there with a crayon in his hand and pointing at the wall. On the white wall was a fairly large drawing. I took a breath and said, "Hmmm." At that point, I had some options. One was to ask how this happened. I chose not to, because it was obvious. The next was to tell him somehow that this was not a good thing. I chose not to say this either because it was clear from him having called me down that he was aware of this. I could have punished him somehow, taken away his crayons, or called his mother, but instead I just said, "Let's see if we can fix this." We, with the help of Grammy, got out the paint, sanded it over, then covered it with some paint, and it was more or less fixed. Drawing on the walls never happened again, and we made sure he always had some paper to draw on. Again, it's not that I liked him drawing on the walls. It could have even been a costly mistake, but it still seems to me that the approach I took was the most effective to not only remediate the situation but to stop it from happening again. The other point here, which I keep coming back to, is my cardinal rule from chapter one: Get on your child's side and stay there. By not punishing Ben and instead spearheading the clean-up effort, it was clear I was here to help him, not harm him. He responded as would most people, with thanks and relief, and even joined in my effort to help.

The second example came from around the same time, again with Ben. California was in the midst of a serious drought at the time and everyone was trying to conserve water. One day we were on the deck and Ben was turning the hose on and off and just watering nowhere. This was not only a waste of water but was like pouring money down the drain. We asked him to stop, with a brief explanation of how water is precious. Ben looked at us and with a bit of a glazed sort of look, turned the hose on, again watering nowhere. At that point, in the face of what some would call clear defiance, there were a number of possible choices. It seems that the most important inward step in this case is to not see this as a personal affront. My sense is this is not how he meant his action. It was more just something he was doing that seemed fun or interesting at the time, and he had a plan to keep the water on. The plan was already worked out in his "mind" and the action of turning on the hose just kind of followed. In any case, we didn't take it personally. Lynda just calmly went over, got the hose, and hung it up on the wall. Again, Ben never wasted water again that either of us ever saw. My point here is that just because you don't use punishments or rewards doesn't mean you have to tolerate behaviors you find unacceptable.

Rather, if we see things from the perspective of the child, the actions usually make sense and are just things to either discuss or, depending on the age of the child, calmly correct. Drawing on walls does seem like an interesting thing to do. The walls are white, they take color well, and it's kind of fun. It just doesn't work for the family or the house. This seemed like an easy point to get across. The thing that doesn't work is to make this a battle of wills. Then it's no longer about drawing on the walls; it's about who has the strongest will. My sense is engaging in a battle of wills with a young child is almost always a losing proposition. Avoid it in any way possible.

The final example is one in which the temptation to use rewards seemed great at the time, but my guess is it would have been harmful and counterproductive. This event happened last year when we were visiting Ben and Sam in New Hampshire. My daughter was moving house that week and we offered to take the boys to a lake house in the area to give her more time to get the new house ready. The boys were mostly with us, and their mom came and went during the week. They were also excited to sleep in their new house. On the last night, we met my daughter and a few friends for an early dinner, and then my daughter said she was going off to make the final touches on the house and that she would see us tomorrow morning. Sam, about four years old at the time, somehow had the idea that he was going to sleep in the new house that night instead of coming back with us to the lake house. When he found out this was not the case and his mother had gone, he felt angry and betrayed. He basically refused to get in the car, and then, once finally in the car, screamed—loudly—from the moment he got in the car. It was horrible for the three of us. Neither Lynda nor I knew exactly how this had come to pass, and Sam was in no position to listen to explanations. This was a time when previously I would have offered some sort of "reward" to calm the situation down. Instead, in spite of the screaming, I did what we had been doing while in the car the whole week, which was to tell a Robin Hood story. The lake we were staying at was in a forest called Sherwood Forest, which is what prompted me to tell the Robin Hood stories whenever we were driving that week. I was a big fan of Robin Hood stories and knew many of them by heart and could make up others. Both Ben and Sam loved the stories and generally asked lots of questions about Robin, Little John, and their many antics. So, even with Sam screaming, I told the story of how Robin disguised himself as a half-blind beggar to win the king's archery contest. As the story went on, Sam's screaming got quieter, presumably so he could hear better. By the middle of the story, he was still clearly upset, but the screaming had stopped.

We got to the lake house, Sam still saying he wanted to go to his new house. We started our outside kickball game and made a fire to roast apple pieces on sticks (a kind of healthy roasted marshmallow variant). By bedtime, he had mostly forgotten about staying in the new house that night, took his shower with Lynda's help, and went to sleep. The next morning, we went to the new house as planned and that seemed to be the end of that incident. The only sequel to report is about a week later, when Sam was again taking a shower, this time while being "supervised" by my daughter, he slipped and banged his knee. He apparently looked at his mom and said with a disdainful tone, "Grammy would have never let this happen." My thought was that this was Sam's retribution for having been wronged by his mom a week earlier.

These, admittedly, are pretty tame examples of "discipline" problems, but my observation over the years is that those who come from an inward stance of punishments and rewards, like many teachers and parents I have seen, have escalating issues to deal with. Those like the two teachers I mentioned earlier, who come from a place of eschewing punishments and rewards, seem to say, "I'm not really sure how I would deal with that kind of disastrous issue because it has never come up." The punishment-and-reward practitioners seem to have disasters come up almost daily. Finding a new approach to "discipline" is an inner practice that accompanies outward change in actions and words. If you focus on the key principle of staying on your child's side, my observation is that your child will remain on your side and be patient with you as you learn these new skills. After all, you are the only parent they get.

For those who are interested in a more in-depth explanation of the repercussions and dangers of using punishments and rewards with children, I would suggest reading Alfie Kohn's book mentioned earlier. There you will find more about the theory, the neurobiology of a rewards-and-punishments-based approach, and practical guidelines for implementing a different approach in your life. The other thing I would strongly suggest, if you are someone, like I was, who struggles with this, is to find a mentor who can help you explore the practice of healthy interaction with children. My guess is that to undertake this change will be one of the most gratifying experiences of your career as a parent.

I would like to finish this chapter with a short recapitulation before we move on to the next section. Thus far, we have been mostly dealing with young children under the age of seven.

In my previous book, *The Nourishing Traditions Book of Baby and Childcare*, cowritten with Sally Fallon, we laid out the case for good nutrition in pregnancy for the mother and in the early years for the child. What we are referring to is a diet based on the principles laid out in *Nourishing Traditions* and re-emphasized in the baby book. We laid out the case for avoiding prenatal ultrasounds (for a more in-depth exploration of the dangers of prenatal ultrasounds, see Appendix 1), routine vaccinations, and the use of fever-suppressing medicines, such as Tylenol or Motrin, in childhood (for more on the dangers of Tylenol, see Appendix 2). We presented the case that to raise children to become healthy adults, they *must* go through childhood febrile illnesses without intervention or only with the intervention of natural medicines. There are no exceptions to this biological imperative. Then, in the first section of this book, I laid out the principles for how the life of the young child can be organized. I clearly don't mean to lay out hard and fast the-child-should-do-this type of rules, but as organizing principles, the young child will thrive in an environment with as much contact with nature as possible and as few extraneous, artificial "toys" as possible. Children thrive and obtain robust health when they are guided through the rhythms of the day, the seasons, and the year.

They learn to trust the safety and beauty of the world around them when they are trusted to find their own activities and when the days have a predictable rhythm. Our job is to provide this rhythm and exposure to the natural world in a safe way. Gardens, forests, rivers, streams, trees, flowers, stones, sand, plants, and insects are your child's best teachers. Let them be in a class with these instructors as much as possible. Then, finally, we touched on some areas where conflict often arises and provided some strategies and concepts for different, more productive ways of dealing with this situation. Underlying all these words is the simple basis for what I believe is the foundation for raising a healthy child: Get on your child's side and stay there, no matter what.

With that, we turn our attention to the older child and the crucial role of school versus education in the raising of a healthy child.

Part II

CHAPTER NINE

School

The three most important books I have ever read in my
life are Dostoyevsky's *Crime and Punishment*, Rudolf
Steiner's lecture series *The Gospel of St. John*, and Ivan
Illich's *Deschooling Society*.

Crime and Punishment showed me that writing can move
another person's soul and shake it to the core. Somehow
after reading that book, I knew I would never be the same
again. I also knew that someday I had to write something
that people might read.

The Gospel of St. John, the first thing I had read of Steiner
at the time and the only book of his that I had available in
Swaziland, showed me that there is a whole different reality, a new way of looking at the world than I had previously
thought. Up until that point, much of the picture I had been
"taught" just didn't make any sense to me at all. Steiner put
things together in a way that suggested that this was largely
because I had been fed a false version of human history.
To begin to see things in a new way was the most exciting
adventure I had ever been on.

Deschooling Society showed me that if I wanted to
understand anything or change anything in our world, I had
to throw off every single assumption I had ever made or ever

been taught to believe. For Illich, even something as universally accepted and seemingly fundamental as the need and benefit of universal schooling must be questioned down to its core. In some ways, this next section is my way of thanking Illich for opening my eyes and allowing me access to a way of questioning that I had never heard before. For that one gift, I am eternally grateful.

There is perhaps nothing in our society that is more universally thought of as "the good" than universal, public, compulsory school for children. While there are some minor disagreements across the political spectrum as to how schooling should be evaluated or paid for, as far as I know, no one is suggesting that the whole phenomenon of universal school is not only a fundamental problem in our culture but in many ways *the* fundamental problem.

Some argue that we should fully fund public education, others that we should make all schools charter schools, but no one is arguing that we shouldn't have school to begin with. How, then, did I come to the conclusion that as long as we are living in a society that mandates compulsory education, there is no possibility of raising a truly healthy child? This includes children who are homeschooled or even unschooled, both of whom suffer from the corrosive effects of living in a schooled society.

To be clear, I am not against learning; I am not against education; I am not even against the presence of some schools. But I will make my case that compulsory education and what is called "the hidden curriculum" of schools is one of the most pernicious influences in our culture. My view is that unless this changes, no political, economic, spiritual, or cultural revolution will bring us the kind of world we all know in our hearts is possible. For that, we must end once and for all the beast of compulsory schooling.

I am going to start to defend what must seem like an unsupportable and wrong-headed perspective by pointing out that I am not alone in coming to this conclusion. Just to give you confidence that this is something we must take seriously, let's hear from some of the most interesting people in our recent past. Let's see what they have to say about "school."

The first quote goes way back to the days before anyone even considered compulsory schooling.

> "Do not train children in learning by force and harshness, but direct them to it by what amuses their minds, so that you may be better able to discover with accuracy the peculiar bent of the genius of each." —Plato

This quote may belong more in the punishment-and-rewards chapter, but it suggests that in order to find the genius in each child, one must be allowed to find out what "amuses" that individual child. This is clearly a far cry from the standardized education of the modern school.

If we fast-forward almost two thousand years, we find a similar sentiment::

> "You cannot teach a man anything; you can only help him find it within himself." —Galileo Galilei

Again, a few centuries later, we find these statements from some of the most important people in the worlds of philosophy, politics, and education:

> "The teacher is a necessary evil. Let us have as few people as possible between the productive minds and the hungry and recipient minds! The middlemen almost

unconsciously adulterate the food that they supply. It is because of teachers that so little is learned, and that so badly." —Friedrich Nietzsche

"Education is an admirable thing, but it is well to remember from time to time that nothing that is worth knowing can be taught." —Oscar Wilde

"What is the purpose of industrial education? To fill the young of the species with knowledge and awaken their intelligence? Nothing could be further from the truth. The aim is simply to reduce as many individuals as possible to the same safe level, to breed and train a standardized citizenry, to put down dissent and originality. That is its aim in the United States and that is its aim everywhere else." —H. L. Mencken

"It is our American habit, if we find the foundations of our educational structure unsatisfactory, to add another story or a wing." —John Dewey

"Schools have not necessarily much to do with education.... They are mainly institutions of control where certain basic habits must be inculcated in the young. Education is quite different and has little place in school." —Winston Churchill

What all these have in common—even coming from the likes of John Dewey, the founder of the American educational system, or Winston Churchill, an arch-imperialist if ever there was one—is that schooling and education/learning are not the same thing. Furthermore, they should not be confused, one for the other, because to do so causes grave harm to the child.

Then, we can turn to the words of perhaps the greatest satirist and writer in American history, Mark Twain, to hear his impressions of "school":

> "I never let my schooling interfere with my education."

> "All schools, all colleges, have two great functions: to confer, and to conceal valuable knowledge."

> "Many public-school children seem to know only two dates—1492 and 4th of July; and as a rule, they don't know what happened on either occasion."

Then, we can hear from diverse modern voices from the worlds of education, business, and politics:

> "Nothing bothers me more than when people criticize my criticism of school by telling me that schools are not just places to learn maths and spelling, they are places where children learn a vaguely defined thing called socialization. I know. I think schools generally do an effective and terribly damaging job of teaching children to be infantile, dependent, intellectually dishonest, passive, and disrespectful to their own developmental capacities." —Seymour Papert

> "Our large schools are organized like a factory of the late nineteenth century: top down, command control management, a system designed to stifle creativity and independent judgment." —David T. Kearns, CEO of Xerox

> "Our present educational systems are all paramilitary. Their aim is to produce servants or soldiers who obey without question and who accept their training as the best possible training. Those who are most successful in the state are those who have the most interest in prolonging the state as it is; they are also those who have the most say in the educational system, and in particular by

ensuring that the educational product they want is the most highly rewarded." —John Fowles, in *The Aristos*

And then, finally, we can hear from Ivan Illich himself on the role of compulsory schooling in modern society:

"School is the advertising agency that makes you believe that you need the society as it is."

"School has become the world religion of a modernized proletariat, and makes futile promises of salvation to the poor of the technological age." (*Deschooling Society*)

"Schools are designed on the assumption that there is a secret to everything in life; that the quality of life depends on knowing that secret; that secrets can be known only in orderly successions; and that only teachers can properly reveal these secrets. An individual with a schooled mind conceives of the world as a pyramid of classified packages accessible only to those who carry the proper tags." (*Deschooling Society*)

"The machine-like behavior of people chained to electronics constitutes a degradation of their wellbeing and of their dignity that, for most people in the long run, becomes intolerable. Observations of the sickening effect of programmed environments show that people in them become indolent, impotent, narcissistic, and apolitical. The political process breaks down because people cease to be able to govern themselves; they demand to be managed." (*In the Mirror of the Past: Lectures and Addresses, 1978–1990*)

Note that this last quote came before the advent of personal computers, cell phones, and other e-devices. Imagine his horror at seeing today's world. And, finally:

"Schools themselves pervert the natural inclination to grow and learn into the demand for instruction." (*Deschooling Society*)

"Schools are even less efficient in the arrangement of the circumstances that encourage the open-ended, exploratory use of acquired skills, for which I will reserve the term 'liberal education.' The main reason for this is that school is obligatory and becomes schooling for schooling's sake: an enforced stay in the company of teachers, which pays off in the doubtful privilege of more such company. Just as skill instruction must be freed from curricular restraints, so must liberal education be dissociated from obligatory attendance. Both skill-learning and education for inventive and creative behavior can be aided by institutional arrangement, but they are of a different, frequently opposed nature." (*Deschooling Society*)

"In fact, healthy students often redouble their resistance to teaching as they find themselves more comprehensively manipulated. This resistance is due not to the authoritarian style of a public school or the seductive style of some free schools, but to the fundamental approach common to all schools—the idea that one person's judgment should determine what and when another person must learn." (*Deschooling Society*)

In the next few chapters, I will try to dissect these statements and attempt to understand the difference between teaching and learning that so many of these people point out. I will attempt to elucidate the hidden curriculum of compulsory schooling so that we can be clear on how it acts as the fundamental impediment to the natural ability of children to learn, grow, and become healthy human beings. Then, I will attempt to help us understand what we parents, grandparents, teachers, and friends can do about this, given the fundamental realities of our current culture. I do understand that our society will not be deschooled any time soon. Even so, there are myriad ways to mitigate the damage. To finish the opening chapter of this section, I want to relate an encounter I had recently with an earnest fellow whom I met at a local farmer's market as he was pursuing his quest for reelection to the San Francisco School Board.

I was walking around the market when a fellow in his mid-forties came up to me to solicit my support for his school board reelection campaign. His main "platform" was to increase educational funding, especially for the "underperforming" schools in San Francisco. Apparently, as in most major cities, there are many such districts, especially in the poorer sections of town. And national, state, and local educational guidelines often punish these schools by giving them less funding.

His point, well taken, is that this is a ludicrous response to poor performance—in essence to make their resources even less. Given the parameters of his argument, I could see no fault in his position. I did want to see if he could see the bigger picture of school and how it has actually degraded the education of the citizens of the country instead of supporting it, as was originally promised. I also made sure not to ask him if he was familiar with Mark Twain's famous comment about school boards: "God made the Idiot for practice, and then He made the School Board."

I started by asking him if he agreed with one of the fundamental premises of our modern public school system—namely, that only through compulsory, mandatory school for all children, no matter their ethnicity, race, or economic status, can we develop an educated citizenry that is able to participate in the experiment we call democracy. He enthusiastically agreed with this premise. This was one of his main arguments for raising the educational level of the more disadvantaged students. I then asked him to name the single most important book ever written that explains the theory and practice of the United States' system of government. He hedged for a moment and when I suggested Thomas Paine's *Common Sense*, he readily agreed. I asked him if he knew how many copies of *Common Sense* were in circulation in the years between 1780 and 1790, during the time of the American Revolution. He didn't know, so I said, according to John Gatto in *The Underground History of American Education*, there were 600,000 copies of this book in circulation as compared to a total population (of "free men") of 2.5 million and another 600,000 "slaves" and other "native" people living in the colonies or new country. If we estimate that each book was read by an average of 1.5 people (I often read my wife's books and vice versa), then probably around 50 percent or more of the citizens in this new country had read the most important book explaining what democracy is all about. Almost none of them had ever been to a school one day in their lives.

In contrast, since he had agreed that one of the main functions of school was to prepare children to participate in the democratic process, and therefore reading this seminal book should be an important part of this education, I asked him to guess how many graduating high school seniors in the San Francisco public school system, from advantaged or disadvantaged neighborhoods, had actually read *Common Sense*. He didn't know but guessed less than 3 percent. I then asked how many graduating students could actually read this book. The word "could" in this context not only means are capable of actually sounding out, i.e., reading the words, but of having the interest, motivation, economic resources, or inclination in any way to read this book that would explain to them the basis of American democracy. He had to admit, with which I agreed, that it would be way less than 1 percent of the graduating high school students. Some surveys show that only about 50 to 60 percent of these students are even literate enough to tackle a complex book such as *Common Sense*. The other 40 to 50 percent basically couldn't care less about American democracy, particularly not if it would interfere with something trending on Facebook.

My final question was: How is it that the very goal you are trying to achieve was met before and without any schooling at all, but now that we have had 150 years of compulsory schooling, virtually no one has any interest in American democracy? How is it that the solution to improving our democracy should be more school, better-funded school, bigger and nicer gymnasiums, etc? As a footnote to this encounter, I happened to check on the outcome of his election. He won handily, except that the real winner, as always in American elections, was the refuse-to-participate vote, which received about 80 percent of the vote in his race, winning by a landslide. Apparently, it is not only children who have been schooled to not give a damn about who makes decisions on their behalf.

On that note, let's begin by examining what has been called the hidden curriculum of our modern, compulsory school system.

CHAPTER TEN

Radical Monopolies:
The Hidden Curriculum

"Radical monopoly," a term I have only seen used by Illich, refers to the situation when one type of activity within a particular area of life comes to dominate the behaviors of the entire society, whether they wish to participate or not. In the business world, it is widely recognized that monopolistic behavior is detrimental to the common welfare because if one company makes all the pots and pans, then in time they will inevitably make poorer quality pots and pans and charge more for them. This is the inevitable consequence of monopolistic behavior in the world of commerce and why "liberal" governments have made a concerted effort to prevent this type of concentration of power in any one activity.

An example of a radical monopoly will demonstrate how corrosive they are to a healthy functioning society populated by healthy, independent, sovereign people. In traditional societies, such as Swaziland, people moved around freely either by walking or by riding in handmade carts. While their top speed was probably 5 to 10 miles per hour, they were all fit and able to move freely around the countryside. Over the years, decades and maybe centuries of using the same paths, the paths were well tended, smooth, safe and easily accessible to everyone. If anyone wanted to move faster, they could attempt to figure out a better cart or maybe even a simple motorized vehicle.

Along came the government, and through the confiscation of people's property (aka taxes) by the threat of violence (putting you in prison), they collected money with which to build high speed roadways all across the country. Then, through this same process of wealth/property confiscation, various government officials were able to purchase Mercedes-Benz vehicles to drive upon these newly built roadways. Inevitably the new roadways, and the speeding vehicles, crisscrossed the traditional walking and cart paths. This made walking and riding in carts along these paths dangerous. The inevitable result was people no longer using these old pathways, so they fell into disrepair. The final result was that, instead of having a population characterized by freedom of movement, we now have a situation in which very, very few people move around at high speeds, while the majority of the people have very restricted movement. They, of course, are angry about this loss of freedom and mobility and start to rebel against the government. The government inevitably responds to this unrest by increasing its military and police force, again paid for by the forceful confiscation of the property of the common people. Before you know it, you have a full-fledged tyrannical state with elite members driving around the country at high speeds in shiny new Mercedes vehicles, while the vast majority of the people are less free, sometimes injured from the vehicles (so, naturally they must build modern hospitals to care for the newly injured), poorer and angry. Welcome to the world of radical monopolies.

Or consider another consequence of the radical monopoly that is otherwise called modern medicine. Imagine, the city of San Francisco has 100 million dollars available to spend on improving the lives of its citizens. Right now, one decision that has been made is that the city hospitals purchase two or three MRI machines to diagnose the occasional brain cancer that is missed on CT scan (an exceedingly rare event) or to help elucidate the anatomy in various sports injuries. This, of course, means that the 100 million dollars will not be used to fix decrepit houses or to put in bike paths or walking lanes that presumably everyone can use. Radical monopolies almost always benefit the rich and accentuate the disparity between the privileged and less privileged in society. They almost always use regressive taxation, meaning the money comes from things like taxes on food or wages, so that not only is it the wealthy who receive most of the benefits from the new MRI machines, but they have somehow swindled the poor into footing the bill. This lunacy, as Illich points out, is one of the primary features of all radical monopolies.

While Illich details many other radical monopolies in our culture these days, by far the most pervasive and destructive is the radical monopoly enjoyed by proponents of mandatory, universal schooling. And, as I pointed out, all radical monopolies are sold to the public as great gifts that no rational human being could or should live without. There are two main components that characterize the insidious, monopolistic nature of universal, compulsory school, which we need to examine carefully. The first, as many of the above quotes point out, is that learning is not the same as being taught, education is not the same as schooling, and wisdom is not the same as having a degree. If you think back to most, if not all, the important skills and attributes in your life, my guess is that very few, if any, were learned in school—skills and qualities like how to speak, to walk, to run, to skip, how to get along with other children or people, how to kiss, how to make love, how to plant a garden, cook your meals, find a good movie, decorate your house, paint the shingles, change the oil in your car, and so on. Most of us, if we really think back on our childhood, actually didn't even learn to read or write in school. It somehow just happened and we have no memory of being taught reading, just as we have no memory of being taught to walk. While I will get more into the actual mechanics of learning to read in a later chapter, I often tell parents who are referred to me because their child is slow in learning to read that, for the vast majority of children, there is one and only one way to prevent them from learning to read by the age of fourteen and that is to teach them when they are not interested. Every other child, with no particular mental handicap, will eventually learn to read fluently as long as it's not forced on them. But again, more on this later.

The insidious nature of schooling, as Plato, Illich, Holt, and others point out, is that school converts the fundamental human desire to learn into an endeavor in which the child must submit to being "taught" at a time and pace of another's choosing. They must learn certain subjects and have no say as to whether they are interested in that particular subject at that time in their lives. They must concentrate on that particular subject for about thirty minutes, at which time they are forced to change to a new subject, again not of their own choosing. They are schooled to think that learning is something that comes from on high, that comes in discrete packages, and that they will be continually graded and evaluated on how competent they become in learning things for which they have no interest and have no relevance to their actual world. As Holt points out, this is a sure-fire way to stifle the natural curiosity and interest in learning that all children bring into the world. In this, it doesn't matter the type of school we are discussing; it's the process of mandatory, compulsory schooling that accomplishes this degradation of the natural curiosity of the child.

Please don't misunderstand me here. I'm not against learning in any way, nor, as I will describe later, am I against any person or any child being taught by someone who knows more about the subject they are interested in. My beef is with the core idea of schooling, which is the fallacious idea that in order to learn, you must be taught, that learning can and should be evaluated or graded, and that any person must subordinate their natural interests to those determined by some unseen bureaucracy that neither they nor their parents have any say in. These are the things that turn the process of learning into the radical monopoly called schooling.

The radical monopoly of schooling undermines the freedom of both the schooled and the unschooled or home-schooled. One of the main consequences of a schooled society, such as we have in the U.S., is that we are told that the path to success—personally, professionally, culturally, and as a society as a whole—is only through school. Here are the words of the former U.S. Secretary of Education Arne Duncan concerning the role of school in our national life:

> America's students have achieved another record milestone by improving graduation rates for a fourth year. The hard work of teachers, administrators, students, and their families has made these gains possible and as

a result many more students will have a better chance of going to college, getting a good job, owning their own home, and supporting a family. We can take pride as a nation in knowing that we're seeing promising gains, including for students of color.

In order to get a good job, in order to achieve social status, in order to participate in democracy, in order to obtain a life that includes security, leisure, and fun, there is one path and one path only and that path is through school. More and more, only a college degree is a reliable pathway to achieving any semblance of the security and meaningful work that we all wish for ourselves and our children. This reality—that in order to have any sort of work in our society, you must be schooled—is so pervasive that even "sanitation engineers" (i.e., garbage collectors) in New York City need to have a high school diploma at the least and soon may need an advanced degree to obtain the job. Don't misunderstand me; I have nothing but admiration for those of us who are willing to collect our garbage. I actually did that one summer and it was no fun. My problem is not with garbage collecting or garbage collectors, but the fact that I see no reason to force these men and women to get a diploma in order to do a job for which this diploma has no relevance or meaning.

The other interesting repercussion of the hidden curriculum of enforced schooling and Duncan's bowing down to the path of schooling and degrees is that if you do the math, you discover that there are currently spots in colleges, junior colleges, community colleges, or other institutions of "higher" learning for about 68.4 percent of high school graduates. If you include the fact that about 84 percent of sixteen- to eighteen-year-olds graduate high school, this means that 49 percent of eighteen-year-olds can go on to get a college degree. There are simply no more spots available for the other 51 percent.

This, of course, means that if these 49 percent of eighteen-year-olds are the winners, then the 51 percent must be the losers. This 49 percent is the approximate limit of the system, as we have no other institutions to confer degrees on the remaining unfortunate citizens. Apparently, we should not be proud of these people. We judge them on their ability to be schooled. As a result, they are seen and unfortunately often see themselves as losers and stupid, instead of the rebellious, creative geniuses that many actually are. But I guess we shouldn't worry too much about these unfortunates, as society does have another radical monopolistic place for them— it's called prison, or prison's cousin, the military.

Radical monopolies, such as the school industry, always rob the less advantaged to support the more advantaged members of society. They often do this in conjunction with related radical monopolies to fleece us of our resources. Consider the taxpayer-funded support conferred on the graduate of a public university with a PhD in finance. After about twenty years of publicly funded school, at a taxpayer expense of about one hundred times the amount spent on the children of the sanitation engineer, they find themselves almost totally without useful life skills. Unlike almost 100 percent of the people in colonial American, or native Americans, or rural Africans, our PhD graduate has no knowledge of how to grow any of his own food and likely no ability to even cook the food he purchases. He is unable to build a house, sew or mend his clothes, most likely only speaks one language and spends the vast majority of his time communicating only with those who have been similarly schooled. His skills and interest in normal human activities have degraded so far that he has even lost interest or doesn't have the time to walk his own dog. This, thankfully, has led to a growth industry in San Francisco called "canine movement specialists." Most such specialists also appear to have advanced degrees, and my prediction is there will soon be courses in the local colleges on the science of canine movement and that one will need a state-supported license and advanced degree in order to supervise canine movement.

The repercussion of our PhD graduate having no useful skills to speak of, in spite of over twenty years of intense schooling, is that the government/corporate conglomerate has had to step in with the introduction of a second radical monopoly in order to find employment for our unfortunate PhD graduate. This second radical monopoly was created when the government/banking/corporate sector created a radical monopoly concerning currency, otherwise known as money. By allowing only one entity in our society to have a monopoly on money creation, money is then magically created out of thin air by the magicians who run our financial institutions. Since none of us lay people understand how money came into being, how financial institutions work, or how to manage our own money, this radical monopoly has created sufficient, highly prized work for those with no useful life skills. Since these tend to be high-paying jobs conferred on people who already had the most societal support in their progress through schooling, the whole gambit pays off for them, as the rich get richer and the poor get fleeced. This is the inevitable consequence of enforced, mandatory schooling and the hidden curriculum it imposes on society.

Illich predicted in the early 1960s that no matter one's political philosophy, no matter whether you are a New Dealer or a trickle-downer, whether you are a communist, capitalist, or any other "ist," if a society goes down the road of compulsory schooling and assigns jobs to those who consume the largest amount of this schooling product, that society will become more and more unequal and polarized. He predicted that, in fifty or so years (from the 1980s), American society would explode in rage, frustration, and futility. He predicted that every society that goes down the path of mandatory schooling will increasingly devour its own resources and become less and less habitable for living beings. Here we are, forty years later, right where he predicted, confronting a mess of epic proportions, and one of the main proposals put forth to right this ship is more schooling for everyone in the world.

A final word here before I turn to what a real learning culture might look like and strategies to help you raise truly educated children who maintain their innate love of learning. I am not trying to blame the PhD graduate. He, like all of us, like me, is a victim of this radical monopolistic system that was conceived in our name. When I woke up in my mid-twenties to realize how incompetent I was, it was a deep source of frustration and rage for me. I felt I had been cheated out of life. I had been cheated out of learning how to be a healthy, full human being, which could and should be the birthright of all people. I have spent the last forty years as a partly futile attempt to re-educate myself or to reconcile myself with the reality that some skills I simply will never acquire. This is a continual source of sadness for me. I am writing this book partly in the spirit of trying to prevent this from happening to your children. It should be possible to raise a child so that at around the ages of sixteen to eighteen, they have all the inner and outer skills needed to create for themselves a useful, meaningful, and joyful life. One of the steps on this road is seeing the beast of compulsory schooling for the radical monopoly that it is.

CHAPTER ELEVEN

Education

Before I get into the educational model I would like to see, which is one of, if not *the* key component of raising healthy children, I would just like to comment on the absurdity of what is apparently a growing trend in our schools these days—namely, the teaching of "tolerance" to school children. Everyone views tolerance, acceptance of others, and a non-judgmental attitude toward our fellow human beings as positive attributes. At least in theory, or at least rhetorically. In fact, most would acknowledge that we live in a fairly racially and ethnically divided culture, one that currently and historically is rampant with intolerance and bigotry. One of the proposals that has been offered to combat this pervasive racism and intolerance is to teach classes on tolerance in schools. Currently, there are many such courses being taught, sometimes to very young children and then again in the high school years. This is an example, however, of the lunacy of having courses on tolerance take place, as they do now, in public schools. Tolerance is about accepting one another's differences, letting others make their own choices out of their own freedom even if you don't agree with the choices made.

Intolerance is about power over another human being, about forcing one's choices, one's point of view on another, regardless of how they feel about or see the choice. Intolerance, and its cousin racism, is about seeing others as "less than" because they are different. We are intolerant because the other has a different skin color, hair color, religious or philosophical view. The question is: How did we come to raise so many millions of people to be outright bigots, intolerant of others with any traits outside of their familiar circle? It starts with school.

No matter if you are teaching a group of six-year-old first graders or sixteen-year-old high school juniors a course on tolerance, the setting is one of forced, mandatory school. The children, collectively, no matter the opinion or thought of the group or of any one particular child, are required to attend for this period of time a "course" on tolerance. They are told—if not directly then through the entire school enterprise—that this is a subject they must learn from a qualified teacher, regardless of the fact that the teacher herself is forcing the children to attend the class. Furthermore, if the first grader does not demonstrate the required level of tolerance at the end of the class, he will often be labeled a "problem" that has to be fixed with more classes on tolerance, or in more extreme cases with psychoactive drugs. This, of course, is done for "their own good," since we cannot tolerate children who don't learn the tolerance lessons they are being taught. The parents are told their child is a problem, will never amount to much, and often must be sent to a tolerance specialist. This person is called by the misleading title of therapist.

For the high school student, the mandatory course on tolerance leads to writing a paper explaining some aspects of how to be a tolerant person or a test that will be graded to make sure the student understands the basic principles of tolerance. If they submit the wrong answers on the test, or turn in an essay that simply states, "Tolerance is bullshit," they will be threatened with a poor grade or even the possibility of not passing or graduating with their class. Flunking tolerance class is simply not tolerated in a respectable society. The consequences of flunking tolerance class are understood by all. Poor grades lead to failure to get into good colleges, leading to poor employment opportunities, leading to homelessness and potentially a life on the streets. Obviously, no parent can tolerate that for their child, so pressure is brought to bear on the recalcitrant student to learn the lessons of tolerance.

Inevitably, what happens is the docile children do well in tolerance class and go on to have academic success. The more independent, rebellious children fail tolerance class and as such are punished unmercifully. My point here is that forced, mandatory schooling, whether the subject matter is tolerance or how to be a bigot, in reality is teaching one thing and one thing only: how to be schooled. No matter if you're teaching capitalism, socialism, communism, or nihilism, if the course happens in mandatory, coerced school, then what you are really teaching is how to be schooled. You are being taught that learning is something that happens in circumscribed packages and is imparted to us by an "expert" in that package. You are being taught that unless you submit to this theory of learning and cooperate fully in its regulations, you are to be shunned, punished, drugged, or relegated to the outskirts of society.

This is the very opposite of the free, independent, courageous healthy human beings who are the goal of raising our children. It doesn't matter if the children in high school English are forced to read Ayn Rand or Karl Marx, what they ultimately learn is that someone has the right to force them to "learn" something against their will and with no regard for their interest or time frame. That is the main lesson they will learn from this type of forced, coercive schooling.

Please understand that I am not against learning about tolerance, nihilism, Ayn Rand, or Karl Marx. My only point, one that I hope everyone will corroborate with their own experience, is that coerced schooling by institutional teachers in any school situation is simply not the way children (or people) learn. That is one of the reasons why in spite of one of the most highly schooled populations in the history of humankind, it is no surprise that we are also extraordinarily intolerant.

Over the past two decades, I have helped to support Sally Fallon in her quest to translate the dietary insights gained from Weston A. Price to the modern world. Price's insights have allowed us to understand that the traditional diet, the diet that produced the healthiest human beings, can be understood to contain three basic components. The first component is full-fat animal foods—foods that help us build our bodily structures. These animal foods include pastured eggs, wild fish and shellfish, grass-fed meats, and pastured, full-fat dairy products. No truly successful human culture exists that didn't include one of these animal foods in their diets. The second component of the traditional diets of the people Price studied are what I call "seed food." This includes grains, beans, seeds, and nuts. Not all, but most traditional peoples include one or more examples of these foods in their diets, always grown as part of an integrated agricultural system, always soaked or sprouted before cooking.

The third component are the plant foods that include vegetables and fruit. The bulk of the traditional diet consists of full-fat animal foods for protein and fat, seed foods for fiber and carbohydrates, and vegetable foods for phytonutrients, vitamins, and minerals. A lunch of kale salad with bean sprouts is not a traditional food lunch. Low-fat dairy products or skinless chicken breast on pasta are not traditional foods; they have no place in the diet of our children if our goal is to raise healthy children.

As I have repeatedly stated, the purpose of this book is not to rehash these dietary principles, as crucial as they may be, but to attempt to shed light on what the life of a healthy child should look like. I bring up Weston A. Price here because while he was not primarily concerned with discipline, school, or the other day-to-day activities of healthy children, he did repeatedly point out how healthy, vigorous, friendly, cooperative, and curious the children of these traditional people seemed to be. He wrote about children who seemed to rarely if ever be sick, children with the complete absence of chronic illness, children who seemed to willingly, even enthusiastically participate in the lives of their families and villages. While he gives few guidelines as to how these children spent their days, between the writings of Price and others and my experience of living in a traditional Swazi village, it has become clear to me that a healthy rhythm of life for a child (ages about three to eighteen), like their diet, includes three parts, four if one includes sleep. If we use this three-part rhythm for a child and combine it with the educational model I am proposing, along with the Price/Nourishing

Traditions dietary guidelines, we will have a great start in our quest to raise healthy children.

Jerry Mander, in his book *In the Absence of the Sacred*, repeatedly points out that almost all traditional peoples spend between eighteen (men) and twenty-three (women—women always have "worked" harder than men) hours per week total on the activities that are done to sustain their lives. These activities include food procurement (hunting, tending the fields, harvesting, weeding, etc.), food preparation, provision of shelter, clothing, transportation, making medicines, killing snakes, and so on. This is the category we could loosely call "work." The things that need to be done to survive and to have an adequate level of ease and comfort in life. That's about two and a half hours per day, max.

The next big category of "activity," which I am not including in my threefold model, is sleep. Generally speaking, traditional people sleep more than modern people, the average being nine to ten hours per day, but this changes according to the seasons, sunlight, and other festivals or events. This leaves about eleven hours per day for non-work activity. As far as I could observe with the Swazis, and from decades of reading about the lives of traditional peoples, the best guess I can make for these eleven hours is that people, including children, mostly "horsed around." There was always a lot of socializing, sitting in small groups telling stories, acting out events of the days, and otherwise spinning yarns of all sorts. They sometimes ate for fun, went for walks, visited neighbors, some went swimming in a nearby river or lake, some sang, danced, or otherwise just kind of hung around. In Swaziland, almost every day the children went for two to three hours with the adults to the fields, where, depending on their age and sex, they either tended the cows, goats, or sheep, helped in the fields with planting, weeding, or harvesting, helped with food preparation, or worked on shelter. Some days, for example, if they thought rain was coming and there was a hole in the roof, they would spend more than the three hours fixing the roof. That was rare. This work part of the day usually took place first thing in the morning and ended before the day's heat.

During the days, the adults mostly gathered in the shade, told stories, and laughed a lot. The children spent the afternoon doing things like playing tag, making old coat hangers into vehicles that they would race around the homestead, doing singing games, or similar activities.

They were almost always outside, almost never with a hat or even with shoes. It seemed to me the only thing they worried about were snakes. Swazis hated snakes for obvious reasons.

If we call this type of activity "play," while remembering that it is in no way purposeless or meaningless, we realize that the bulk of traditional people's waking hours were spent doing this type of play. I propose that this should still be the case, for young and old alike, but that we can add a third type of activity, which adds an educational component to our lives that was at least partially lacking in traditional cultures. This "educational" component optimally can take about one to two hours per day from the "play" time, but no more. Also, just to be clear, I am including meal times in the play section, as this also seemed to be a time when everyone was mostly just enjoying life.

Also, leave aside for a moment the fact that this system I am describing doesn't exist at this point in our culture. My point is it needs to be created for us to get back to raising healthy children. Once you understand the principles, you can begin to organize your child's life around these general guidelines. Then, the more people who join us, the easier it will become. If we don't know where we're going, we can be sure we'll never get there. This one-to-two-hour period per day, with, of course, as much day-to-day, week-to-week, month-to-month flexibility as needed, should be used to cultivate the interests of the child. This is the time when the genius of the individual child should be sought and cultivated. This is the time that distinguishes the modern person from the person in a traditional culture. We live in a new age for humankind, an age of untold potential; this slot in the day is when we cultivate the unique gifts of your child.

Imagine your child is interested in gardening and growing plants. As a parent, this is the time to make every attempt to connect your child with a mentor, a gardener, or a garden of their own so they can explore this interest. The educational world I envision is one in which experienced, expert gardeners are encouraged in many different ways to offer their guidance to interested children. Imagine, then, if in your town or community, there were ten such children of a variety of ages who wanted to learn gardening, or it could be basketball or playing the cello, or discussing Nietzsche's views on freedom, or playing the recorder, or projective geometry, or learning to speak Urdu, or the names of butterflies, or whatever. The people who know these subjects well could offer to meet with the group and could suggest different groups for children of different levels of expertise in the subject. Some might even be just one on one. Imagine, then, your child, who has a clear interest in learning to play dungeons and dragons, getting to meet regularly with a master and potentially a small group of others with a similar interest. There are no grades, no degrees passed out, imagine how "discipline" would work in this situation. If nine of the ten children were completely captivated by the teacher of the game, if one child "acted out," my guess is they would be immediately and completely admonished, not by the teacher but by the other children. I can guarantee that if Steph Curry were teaching a class of ten children who were passionate about learning to shoot a basketball, there wouldn't be a single instance when he would have to punish or reward any child. This is a dream situation, not only for learning but also for teaching.

For those who are concerned that no child would choose to learn basic skills such as math and arithmetic, just imagine that a child who wants to learn to build a tree house, a fort, or whatever, or who wants to learn how to fix cars or airplane engines is told by a master in those fields, "I can't teach you to build if you don't know basic math." I imagine that child would go home to their parents and demand that someone teach them basic math right now. Not in the three to six years it takes to learn in school, but in three weeks, he would want to be competent enough in math to go back to do the building class. Illich in his "school" in Guatemala proved that you could teach almost 100 percent of illiterate peasants to read fluently in six weeks, but only if the "goal" of learning to read was to understand the contracts these people had with their landlords who were trying to rip them off.

Again, an educational culture such as I am describing would use modern administrative techniques to help bring children with a particular interest together with someone who can help them understand and even master that subject. This could include everything from one session on how to plant carrots to a series of conversations about the use of symbolism in the plays of Pirandello to a year-long course in projective geometry. The rules of this educational culture would include that no degrees are given, no preference for jobs are given to those who consume a certain amount of schooling, but rather that people are "hired" to be part of the city's symphony orchestra or to care for the gardens of a local senior center based solely on their competence and ability to perform the job.

If the child can learn projective geometry or classical cello without a single lesson or class, that's fine. For most, a robust educational culture would provide children of all ages with the ability to find and cultivate their own individual genius. I fully understand that this is not the culture we currently live in and my intention is not to create despair for those who see no possibility to raise their children in this fashion, no matter how much they agree with the basic principles. I would only point out that when *Nourishing Traditions* came out and the Weston A. Price Foundation began over twenty years ago, it was almost impossible to find kombucha, pastured eggs, grass-fed meat, coconut oil, raw milk, sauerkraut, bone broth, or many of the other staples of a traditional diet for most Americans. Now you can order online, or purchase in almost any city in the country, a wide variety of all these products. We will someday have to become an educational culture or, as Illich pointed out, we will perish in a flurry of rage and destruction. I am presenting a starkly different model than the college-for-everyone, school-as-salvation model. Again, if you don't know where you are going, you'll never get there. With that said, let's look at some possible options for those in a variety of situations to implement these changes today.

The first scenario is for those who currently live or plan to live on a homestead that is fundamentally modeled on subsistence living. These families attempt to grow as much of their food as possible, and make as much of their heat, energy, "products" (like soap, clothes, etc.) as possible. For them, it's only a matter of facilitating (never forcing) the children to participate in the business of the homestead for a few hours each day. The vast majority of children love to do "useful" things, especially if they involve animals, gardens, splitting wood (age appropriate), building chairs, or those sorts of things. Then, for a good chunk of the day, the children can be on their own, hopefully either by themselves or with "gangs" of other friends or neighbors. The addition for this family is that a serious effort can and should be made to find any special interests this child may have. You may have to expose them to all sorts of activities to find the one(s) that resonate, but that is your role in this scenario. Once you find their particular interest, see what you can do to make it happen. For older children, they can also be in charge of finding and making these types of classes, encounters, or events happen; for younger children, they will need your help.

The next scenario is for suburbanites or city dwellers who have little to no access to subsistence activities. For these children, there is a "school" option I will discuss in the next chapter that can be counted as the two-to-three-hour "work" component of their day. While this will involve some modification of the school schedule and doesn't address the problem of the tyranny of degrees as a prerequisite for employment, it does constitute an improvement in your child's life. This school rhythm is actually the norm for many places in Europe. The children go to school from 9 a.m. to 12 p.m. Then they are home to pursue their own interests or no interests at all.

Don't be afraid to let you child be "bored." Most people in traditional cultures spent a fair amount of time just walking around, sitting around, or doing other "non-productive" activities. Often this is when the most profound ideas are hatched. In this scenario, the other component, the one to two hours per day, also becomes crucial as school may not be providing an outlet or exposure to their unique interests. Again, the more the entire culture becomes an educational culture, the easier it will become to help children find unique outlets for their interests.

The final scenario is for those parents who, because of their economic circumstances, job requirements, or personal situations, seemingly have no choice but to send their children to full-time public schools and often other "care" situations after school. For those children, who in many ways risk becoming victims of the radical monopoly of school, my most important suggestion is to do whatever is in your power to be your child's advocate as they navigate this system. Don't let anyone suggest or tell your child they are stupid, lazy, or otherwise inadequate.

That suggestion, along with getting your child out into whatever nature setting is possible for you as much as possible, may be the best you can do at this point. And, as I keep emphasizing, get on your child's side, look for every opportunity to nurture your child's uniqueness, no matter who or what authority you must confront. Your child will see this and you will have a life-long ally. In many ways, this profoundly loving attitude toward your child is the most powerful step you can take in your quest to raise a healthy child in our toxic world.

Our next step is to look into the world of Waldorf education along with what many would call the primary educational imperative of school, which is learning to read. In this exploration, we also find some surprising insights that have much to teach us about the process of raising healthy children.

CHAPTER TWELVE

Learning to Read

Probably many of you have seen the bumper sticker that says, "If you can read this, thank a teacher."

Whenever I bring up or discuss the idea of deschooling society, people tend to always come back with the fear that unless children are taught in school to read, we will end up with a completely illiterate society. No matter how much I point out that the literacy rate for reading books like *Common Sense* was actually higher before anyone went to school than it is now, this fear of illiteracy is something that people just can't seem to overcome. In light of this, it is worthwhile exploring Rudolf Steiner's view on learning to read and his whole conception of educating children as a kind of counterweight to the modern hysteria surrounding reading. This became especially poignant to me as I recently had a patient whose child was entering first grade in a local public school and was required, before being allowed to enter the class, to be able to read one hundred words. The parents know a little about my views on reading and schooling, so they politely declined my offer to teach him some words. I imagine, rightly so, they might have been worried about which words I would have chosen to teach him.

To be clear, just as in my previous books I don't present Steiner's ideas as being some sort of gospel that we all must blindly follow. On the other hand, this guy wrote the curriculum for arguably the most successful school movement on the planet. He came up with all the medicines for an entirely new system of medicine. He gave the directions for a cancer medicine, mistletoe, which is far and away the most successful natural medicine for cancer in current use. He gave the directions for an agricultural system, biodynamics, that has transformed the agricultural landscape in the world, in particular in the world of viticulture. He was an architect, sculptor, scholar of Goethe, founder of a new art of movement and color therapy—and those were only a few of his accomplishments. It would seem that, at least, we might want to hear him out and be very sure that his perspective is not valid before it is dismissed out of hand.

Here is what Steiner had to say about learning to read:

> But all the things that we are usually advised to do with kindergarten children are quite worthless. The things that are introduced as kindergarten education are usually extraordinarily "clever." One is, I might say, quite fascinated by the cleverness of what has been thought out for kindergartens in the course of the nineteenth century. The children certainly learn a great deal there, they almost learn to read. They are supplied with letters of the alphabet, which they have to fit into cut out letters and such like. It all looks very clever and one can easily be tempted to believe that it really is something suitable for children, but it is of no use at all. It really has no value whatsoever, and the whole soul of the child is spoilt by it. Even down into the body, right down into physical health, the child is ruined. Through such Kindergarten methods, weaklings in body and soul are bred for later life.*

---

* Rudolf Steiner, *The Kingdom of Childhood*, p. 18.

Or later from the same lecture:

> People will object that the children then learned to read
> and write too late. This is only said because it is not
> known today how harmful it is when the children learn
> to read and write too soon. It is a very bad thing to
> be able to write early. Reading and writing as we have
> them today are really not suited to the human being till
> a later age, in the eleventh or twelfth year, and the more
> one is blessed with not being able to read and write
> well before this age, the better it is for the later years
> of life. A child who cannot write properly at thirteen or
> fourteen (I can speak out of my own experience because
> I could not do it at that age) is not so hindered for later
> spiritual development as one who early, at age seven or
> eight, can already read and write perfectly. These are
> things that the teacher must notice.[*]

When my daughter started fifth grade in the Waldorf
school, she got a new teacher because the old one left (usually the teacher stays with the children from grades 1 to 8
in Waldorf schools). The new teacher was my next-door
neighbor, and within a week or so of starting the new year,
I got a call from the teacher asking me if I knew that my
daughter couldn't read. I called her over, showed her one of
the books we had, and she recited it perfectly. Then when
I asked her what this word was, she had no clue. I don't
think she could have read "run, Spot, run" at that time. She
could, however, plant a garden, knit hats and scarves, sing,
play recorder, speak some French, and many other things.
She was overall happy and just completely not interested in
reading. When I called her teacher back, I had one request
and that was to ensure that in no way was she to feel bad,

---

[*]   Ibid., pp. 26–27.

stupid, or somehow lacking because she didn't read. I left it up to his judgment whether to help her with reading or not.

By the end of the year, she decided to read *The Mists of Avalon*, which I must confess I gave her without reading it myself, thinking it was a book about King Arthur and the women of the court. After reading it, I could see how a young girl discovering this book would quickly teach herself to read. Steiner's educational philosophy centers around the idea that just as the human being's body has evolved, so too has his consciousness. He lays out a scenario, confirmed by almost all the initiates throughout history (see, for example, *The Secret History of the World* by Mark Booth) that human consciousness has also evolved through the ages.

Starting with a dreamier, less individualistic "mind," the evolving human being has through the eons developed an awareness or consciousness more centered around clear thinking and a heightened sense of his own individuality. In Steiner's pedagogy, he taught that each child, to be truly educated to unfold their unique destiny, should undergo a recapitulation of the history of humanity. Starting from the dreamy, imitative consciousness of the pre-school years through the gradual coming to awareness of the years between the change of teeth and puberty, the Waldorf curriculum meets the child at each of these stages. The child in the first few grades is exposed to fairy tales, stories of bravery and valor, as they themselves progress inwardly through these stages of life. At nine years old, they begin to cross the bridge from the consciousness of a child to the awake awareness of a young adult. This evolution progresses until they step into the fully awake adult consciousness at around age twenty-one. Human beings started to read in this evolutionary process at around the eleven-to-twelve-year mark of our development. Forcing children to read earlier shifts their awareness in a way that Steiner postulates will have negative repercussions for their entire lives. This is a powerful picture of the way the education of the child for freedom and for an unfolding of their unique destiny can be approached. It is also the only argument that I have ever heard that helps the phenomena of school make sense for me.

However, and this is a major barrier, even Waldorf schools in our time do not and cannot overcome the hidden curriculum that is the foundation of our mandatory schooled society. Even Waldorf schools must confront the fact that they are also enforcing a hidden agenda on their children. And, as time has gone on, it is the rare Waldorf school that discourages reading and writing until age eleven or twelve and that doesn't end up spending considerable effort preparing children for the tests and requirements needed to be consumers of more schooling.

To be clear, it's not that I am proposing that we prohibit or somehow stop our children from learning to read and write before age eleven or twelve. Rather, we understand that a healthy child should have most of the life skills in place by that time, the skills that virtually all human beings at age twelve before our current Industrial Age could easily manage. A fully educated child at age twelve can and should be competent in all the skills needed to run their own homestead. In addition, they can usually manage to have good social skills, be competent on at least one musical instrument, know at least one other language, and have some sense of where their special interests lie. This is what we should consider normal for a twelve-year-old in our time. This sometimes happens with children currently in Waldorf schools or those who are unschooled or homeschooled on the family homestead. It is only when we cripple the young child with a reading-only mentality that they become disadvantaged in regard to their skill acquisition and creative development. This is not the sign of a healthy child. Rather, as so many authors have suggested, it is the path to a schooled mind, fit only to be a consumer in a culture that devours the earth. It is for this reason that for our children before age twelve, it is these life skills that should be the entire focus of our educational efforts. If they want to teach themselves to read along the way, if they realize that to build a rocket ship out of cardboard, they need to read the manual, then so be it. We just don't help them any more than is absolutely necessary.

Insofar as modern Waldorf schools stay true to or return to this vision and mission, they seem like the most reasonable option, particularly if they could move to only having hours from nine till noon.

But while Steiner himself clearly had outstanding ideas about the raising of children, the development of children, and the stages of learning that children go through, unfortunately there was a fatal flaw built into the fabric of the Waldorf school movement. Simply put, embedding this view of child development into a *school* setting ensured that Waldorf schools would develop the same tyrannical tendencies found in all schools. There is no clearer proof of this than examining the policies of literally all the Waldorf schools in the US during "Covid," as they embraced the same anti-scientific and authoritarian policies concerning "distance learning," masks, "social distancing," and all the other policies found in the entire school system, both public and private. Sometimes using the excuse of "if we don't, they'll close us down," the schools uniformly chose to conform to the dictates of the state rather than protect and nurture the children in their care. Again, this is the predictable trajectory that comes from being a "school."

While Steiner may not be 100 percent correct in his dire warnings about the repercussions of premature intellectual development, he is not to be ignored either. If you ever have the opportunity to meet children raised in the manner I am speaking about, see what you think, try to understand the qualities you are experiencing in this human being. Answer for yourself if this is what we can mean by raising a healthy child in our toxic world.

Chapter Thirteen

Electronic Devices

Some time ago, I watched the testimony of an internist from Michigan in front of the U.S. Senate committee responsible for agreeing to the 5G rollout across the U.S. She was clearly a bit nervous speaking in front of these senators for her allotted ten minutes, and also clearly frustrated that she was only given such a short time slot to present her years of research. In these ten minutes, armed with a stack of papers on her desk about two feet high, she made the case over and over again that the science concerned with the biologically harmful effects of 4G frequencies on *all* life forms, but in particular in the developmental stages of plants, animals, and humans, is profound and "settled science." In other words, exposure to 4G electromagnetic frequencies negatively impacts growth and development, damages the integrity of the various tissues of the body across all species, creates distortions of cell division and growth, produces adverse effects on behavior and socialization across all species, and does all of this with the dose–response relationship typical of biological toxins. The more the exposure, the worse the damage. This is with the weaker 4G network currently in place. She emphasized over and over that this should be considered "settled science" and that there are virtually no investigators in this field who have come to a different conclusion (see Appendix 1 for a description of the current research on the deleterious effects of EMF exposure).

In her brief time slot, she then presented evidence that the planned 5G rollout would create an exponential increase in the harmful biological effects to our cells, tissues, disease incidence, and social/emotional parameters, and that the scope of these negative effects can still only be imagined or extrapolated at this point. What we know for sure is bad enough. What we don't yet know might be many times worse. She, and others, have likened the effects of 4G exposure on our children to having each three-year-old smoke two packs of cigarettes a day. If someone proposed this, they would be derided as a madman. Yet there, in the "hallowed" halls of the U.S. Senate, these leaders in our society calmly debated the timing and economic consequences of rolling out an exposure that makes cigarette exposure look like eating a bit too much honey in your diet.

My question is how and why is this even up for debate? If you discover a substance or exposure that irreparably damages the tissues of young children, and you can prove it beyond a shadow of a doubt, how did this become something of which we debate the merits? Seriously, what is wrong with us?

Over the past few decades, I have generally considered that the two most damaging radical monopolies we live with are mandatory schooling, with degree acquisition being a prerequisite for economic or social "success," and the radical monopoly of currency creation. Currency creation concentrates wealth in the hands of a few, inexorably placing immense power in these few hands; mandatory schooling allows this economic inequality to be accepted and makes achieving the state of excessive currency acquisition a goal of the common person. All the other radical monopolies—medicine, transportation, and so on—fall in line behind these two. Recently, I have had to revise these conclusions. There is a third radical monopoly that is rapidly overtaking and even surpassing the damage done by the first two, and that is the radical monopoly of electronic devices.

There are two interrelated components of the radical monopoly of electronic devices. The hallmark of all radical monopolies is that they adversely impact not only those who participate in them but also those who don't. If you use the resources of an "undeveloped" country to build paved roads for high-speed automotive traffic over the previously used walking paths, not only will the elites in that society who have the resources to buy Mercedes be the only ones who use the road (this was exactly the situation in Swaziland) but the bulk of the people can no longer use the pathways to walk or ride their bicycles because the roads have become unsafe for pedestrians. In this way, it becomes a radical monopoly, and the "development funds" used to build roads actually degrade the health and quality of life of the vast majority of the citizens of that society.

The two components of the radical monopoly of electronic devices are first that the infrastructure that is built to support these devices—i.e., the 4G and soon the 5G network—is useful only for those with the resources to own such a device, but are profoundly toxic to all, whether they use the device or not. No matter where you live, no matter your profession, your political views, no matter whether you understand or even care about the science, your children are being harmed by exposure to the electronic infrastructure—you have no choice in the matter. That is the very definition of a radical monopoly. And if something dramatic is not done, it's about to get much, much worse.

The second and in some ways more widely recognized component of this radical monopoly is that electronic devices, all of them, are meant to addict your child to an experience of the world that is not grounded in real, personal exposure to the natural world. No matter what you are "watching" or "interacting" with on a screen, you are only being exposed to a tiny sliver of the richness of a tree, a garden, a friend, or even a baseball bat. This is particularly damaging and poignant for a child, whose main focus in their development is how to learn to interact with and understand the richness and possibilities in our world. The user of electronic devices is inexorably and without exception impoverished in their experience of the world, no matter what they are seeing on the screen. That basic concept should be clear to anyone who makes the effort to consider the consequences of screen experience as compared to actual experience of the world.

Furthermore, as is very clearly outlined in Nicanor Perlas's book *Humanity's Last Stand* and openly described in many other places, the developers and engineers who work at places like Apple, Google, Microsoft, Facebook, Instagram, Pinterest, and many others have whole divisions in their companies devoted to creating techniques to make users addicted to their devices. They use hidden messages, streaming devices, pop-ups, and more to clearly and openly make people, and in particular children, crave the further use of their device. Again, of this there is no doubt; it's part of the business model, spoken about quite openly without any sense that it is anything but business as usual.

What makes electronic devices into radical monopolies, besides the harmful effects of the actual network that is built to support these devices, is that once electronic devices become embedded in the culture of children, any child without access to the use of these devices and the social media platforms they support becomes ostracized and is often considered a "loser."

Essentially this means that all but the most independent minded of our children will find themselves with no choice but to begin to be consumers of electronic devices. This is reenforced in schools that, in many cases, require the use of these devices to complete required assignments. Even the reluctant child, finding left out of the general social life of his peers, teased and shunned, will break down and demand a devise. Once they start, as we all have experienced, the planned addictive effects kick in, and the child is well on his way to something that neither he nor you intended.

I raised my children in an era before electronic devices, so I never had to face this tragic situation in my own life as a parent. In working with this as a doctor, friend, and grandparent, the conclusion I have reluctantly come to is that like all radical monopolies, and in many ways to a greater extent than with other examples, it is not in your power as a parent to eliminate the harmful effects of electronic devices on your child. This is a social, political, and economic issue and will need to be addressed collectively; the power of the individual is limited, but it is not zero. I point this out in my attempt to help you find the road between the Scylla of feeling hopeless and powerless, on the one hand, and the Charybdis of feeling paralyzed by guilt and shame, on the other, as you find yourself inevitably compromising your own values. Also, in my experience, the strategy I outlined in the chapter on solving the issue of food fights doesn't seem to work for resolving the modern battle between parents and children over electronic devices. They are simply too addicting for the children, so the strategy of giving them autonomy in this realm often spirals into further battles. With that said, here are my suggestions for at least mitigating the insidious influence of electronic devices on your child.

First, I would involve yourself in whatever local campaigns are happening in your community to stop the introduction of smart meters, the 5G network, cell tower placement, and any other attempts to enlarge the infrastructure underlying electronic devices. It's hard to say if this has any hope of success, but lately there have been a few minor victories. Second, in your own home avoid installing any wireless system, and if you must use electronic devices, use them only on wired systems that go through your phone line. Third, in your own life use electronic devices, social media, and the like as little as possible. When you have decided this is as little as you can possibly use these devices in our current world, go down by another third and that should be about right. Fourth, turn off the electricity to your bedrooms, or at least the bedroom of the children in your house, at least one hour before bedtime. They and you can use candles for reading, talking, and telling stories. Fifth, there are a variety of devices that are currently being sold that claim to mitigate at least some of the damage done by exposure to EMFs. I have no idea which ones are best or whether any of them really work, but in any case, I have one such device in every room of my house and at least one on every device or appliance in my home and office.

And, finally, if electronic devices are truly as harmful as all the current research seems to suggest, and if they are deliberately being engineered to addict our children to their use, and if Steiner is correct that children should be "raised" in a way that recapitulates the evolution of humanity, then there is no other conclusion that any rational person can come to as concerns the use the electronic devices for children. That conclusion is that before the age of eighteen, they should be completely avoided. Limiting, regulating, making deals about, bargaining for a certain amount of screen time for a child will inevitably set you up for a lifetime of battles with a high percentage of children, and you will lose this battle. I am fully aware that this is completely impossible for most of us; that is tragic in itself, but do the above strategies, hold out as long as you can, do everything possible to enrich and enliven your child's contact with the real world, help them cultivate a network of friends who will join them in avoiding electronic devices, and finally tell the teacher, if your child is in school, that the dog ate Johnny's cell phone (it goes without saying, though, that this wouldn't be very good for your dog). If, as in an example I recently heard, your child's teacher insists that your child turn in their papers or assignments written on a computer instead of by hand, say, "Fine," and then the next day bring them a glyphosate popsicle and say, "My child will turn this in electronically as soon as you finish eating this popsicle" (or you might want to find a new school). Your child will be happier, healthier, and if we are lucky, will experience this themselves and join you, even push you, for a life free of electronic poisons.

CHAPTER FOURTEEN

Returning to Life

So far, I have attempted to make the case that your child is a unique and gifted human being who deserves to be treated as such. I have attempted to describe some of the basic principles to use in raising children in general, such as a nourishing diet, avoiding vaccines, shepherding them through common childhood illnesses, time spent in nature, a healthy rhythm of the day, and many others. In addition, I have repeatedly tried to make the case that your child is also a unique being with distinct needs, interests, talents, and weaknesses. This is particularly important in deciding how to implement an "educational" program for your child, a program that brings out the genius inherent in all of us. I also tried to warn against the many current radical monopolies that either injure or restrict the freedoms of all, whether we are users of the system or not. The current compulsory school system is one of the primary examples of this type of radical monopoly, and I attempted to make my case that it must be dismantled down to its core for us to be able to create a culture that truly honors the gifts of all children. In the following chapter, I will try to lay out some of the principles on which a new educational society can be built, and how this will serve to free up the energies and creativities of young and old alike.

The nagging question I wish to address in this chapter is: What is the basis or foundation for this suggested individuality and uniqueness of your child? After all, one prevailing model of human development is that although we enter the world with a unique genetic make-up, we are basically blank slates who must be educated (i.e., schooled) to become fully valuable and functioning members of society; without this intensive schooling process, we will never become fully contributing members of society. Guidelines will be drawn up, goals will be presented as far as skill acquisition by the various ages in the child's life, punishments and rewards will be suggested for those who either successfully meet these guidelines or for those who fail. Underneath it all is the theory that unless we diligently school our children to become productive citizens, these blank slates will be filled with destructive or non-productive ideas or actions. But what if the "blank slate" theory is simply not true? What if our children come into the world with something more akin to a "spiritual intention," and rather than being the ones who decide what is right and good for our child, our real job is to recognize and encourage the unfolding of this unique being who has been placed in our care? Could it be that the "blank slate" theory is just that, an unproven and unfounded conception of the human being that needs to be replaced as soon as possible?

Starting about five decades ago, the University of Virginia, under the guidance of Ian Stevenson, established the Division of Perceptual Studies, whose mission is to rigorously study and document cases of children around the world who report memories of past lives. In recent years, this work has been taken over by Jim Tucker, MD, who is the Bonner-Lowry Associate Professor of Psychiatry and Neurobehavioral Sciences at the University of Virginia. Between these two men, they have published in peer-reviewed journals over a thousand rigorously studied cases of young children, usually between the ages of three and six, who have clear and verifiable memories of past lives.

Dr. Tucker has written two books on this subject—*Life before Life: A Scientific Investigation of Children's Memories of Previous Lives* and *Return to Life*—both of which go into great detail about the case studies they are presenting. In these books, Dr. Tucker presents his evidence that the experiences of the children he is presenting have only one possible explanation: they, or some "part" of them, had a previous life experience that is still active and relevant in their current life. Everyone interested in these fascinating cases is encouraged to read both of these books in their entirety, as I can only give a brief glimpse into these stories, some of which run for forty pages in the book. Dr. Tucker, in the final chapter of *Return to Life*, gives a clear and cogent explanation of how these phenomena might arise. His explanations are perfectly consistent with the discoveries of mystics throughout history. Simply put, consciousness is first; consciousness is *before* matter. There is nothing behind awareness or consciousness, and substance or matter is best conceived of as "congealed" consciousness.

All matter, including our current body, is just a congealed electromagnetic field; physical particles are only a model with no proven existence. Your child, whether they remember it or not, whether you agree with it or not, whether you will discover any of the details or not, is unique because they have a past. This past is one of the relevant factors that has inspired their individuality in this life and is the underlying picture of why it is so crucial that all of us in a position to help raise a child see it as our primary responsibility to help them discover, honor, and fulfill their unique destiny.

Again, I only want to give some very brief details of two of Dr. Tucker's cases to hopefully pique your interest in further exploring this subject. The first was the story of a young boy who, starting around age three (the usual time these memories seem to emerge), became obsessed with golf. Neither his parents or anyone else in his world had any contact with golf, and his first exposure was seeing someone hit a golf ball on TV as his father was scrolling through the channels. As time went on, and no one in his family gave him any golf clubs or balls, he would fashion sticks and little balls and play golf on his own. He kept pestering his parents, and, finally, they started taking him to a driving range to hit real golf balls with a real golf club. Somewhere along the way, an older golf professional noticed that his golf swing bore an uncanny resemblance to the swing of Bobby Jones, one of the greatest golfers of all time. The parents started showing their child pictures of different people and the child could not only clearly identify Bobby Jones in pictures, claiming that was "me," but could correctly identify many members of Bobby Jones' extended family. At some point, the parents contacted Dr. Tucker to see what he thought of this situation; some more rigorous testing ensued.

As the children get older, they often begin to realize that having these kinds of experiences makes them "weird," so according to Dr. Tucker, one must be careful in how these children are approached. That said, there are ways they have developed over decades of research with similar children to get at the facts of each case.

For example, they showed this child a series of houses. In each case, the child could correctly identify the house that Bobby Jones lived in as opposed to pictures of similar houses that Bobby Jones had no known contact with. He could reliably pick out many of the friends, relatives, even fellow golfers from Bobby Jones' era out of a lineup of similar-looking people. In his play, this child could construct the original design of the Augusta National Golf Course, a course that Bobby Jones had a major part in designing. He correctly placed water hazards, sand traps, tee boxes, and other distinguishing features on the correct holes even though he had never been anywhere near Georgia and as far as the parents knew had never seen pictures or computer images of this site. Of course, we should all be wary of these types of claims; it's certainly possible the parents somehow put him up to these stunts for potential economic gain. The problem with this conclusion is that it's very hard to believe this if you read the entire case study, and this University of Virginia program has compiled thousands of such cases from all over the world. If this is a giant hoax, it's an extraordinarily well-planned, well-executed strategy for seemingly no purpose.

Interestingly, as is usual in these cases, by around the age of seven, most of the child's ability to remember the details of the life of Bobby Jones receded. However, at last count, the child had won about 95 percent of the golf tournaments he had entered, even when matched against much older competitors. Somehow, like a young Mozart of golf, this child came into the world with a clear destiny and a clear calling.

Somehow, it's hard for me to imagine that there is a gene or a group of genes that code for this extraordinary talent or that are responsible for these memories.

The second story has many similar characteristics to all the stories in Dr. Tucker's books. This one involves a child of similar age who, like many of these children, became obsessed with a certain subject or event. Bearing a lot of similarity to the experience of people with PTSD (post-traumatic stress disorder), the child was continually playing with airplanes and talking about airplanes that were crashing into the ocean. This was clearly a traumatic experience for the child, and the growing obsession with airplanes and crashes ultimately led the parents to contact Dr. Tucker's group. As time went on, again as is usual in these cases, the child started to remember more and more details about the plane crash he kept referencing. He gave great details of the plane involved, could pick it out of a lineup of similar types of planes, and knew uncanny details about the configuration, engine type, and flight mechanics of this type of plane. Eventually, as the parents and researchers began to piece together the story, linking it to events in the Pacific theatre of World War II, they could make reasonable guesses as to the actual people involved and how the actual event of the plane crash and subsequent death of the copilot actually happened. In each case, when they showed the child a lineup of possible subjects, the child could correctly pick out the copilot that had died in the crash, who had the same name the child called himself during times of distress. He knew the location of the copilot's home and could also pick out his house and family members from a lineup of similar houses and people.

Again, as time went on, most of the memories faded but not the interest in aviation and the exploration of plane crashes and other aviation mishaps.

Reading these and many other stories is something we should all experience. To consider the fact that these are actually true stories but for some reason are only accessible in certain cases—often cases in which some overwhelming trauma has occurred—is to be forced to reexamine our conception of life and the children who are entrusted to our care. Clearly, I am not suggesting we understand exactly what is happening here or the mechanism for how these types of memory-transfers happen. Maybe there is some sort of collective unconsciousness as Jung suggested. Maybe there is a law of reincarnation as described by Rudolf Steiner. Whatever the case may be, these stories are a clear refuting of the "blank slate" theory. Your children are not blank slates for you to mold into productive citizens. They are spiritual beings having an experience, perhaps one of many, in a physical form. Or, as the Nobel-Prize-winning neurophysiologist Sir John C. Eccles states:

> I maintain that the human mystery is incredibly demeaned by scientific reductionism, with its claim to account for all of the spiritual world in terms of patterns of neuronal activity. This belief must be classified as a superstition. We have to recognize that we are spiritual beings with souls existing in a spiritual world as well as material beings with bodies and brains existing in a material world.

Or, in the words of the famous theoretical and mathematical physicist Roger Penrose:

My position on consciousness demands a major revolution in physics.... I've come to believe that there is something very fundamental missing from current science.... Our understanding at this time is not adequate and we're going to have to move to new regions of science.

And, finally, the words of Nobel Laureate and father of quantum physics Niels Bohr:

We can admittedly find nothing in physics and chemistry that has even a remote bearing on consciousness.... Quite apart from the laws of physics and chemistry, as laid down in quantum theory, we must also consider laws of quite a different kind.*

We must realize that our children come with strengths, weaknesses, intentions, fears, goals, and a path. It is our job, in our quest to raise healthy children, to honor and, as far as possible, to understand this unique path. This doesn't mean grilling children about past lives; it means simply asking yourself the question from time to time: Who is this child? How can I help him fulfill his destiny? That is your primary job as a parent.

---

* All quotes from "The One Mind," an article by Larry Dossey, MD, in *Tikkun*, fall 2018.

CHAPTER FIFTEEN

Envisioning a World
Fit for Our Children

In ancient times, human beings had a different consciousness than they do today. These humans, some of whom,
until recently, were still extant in the various tribes of the
world before any contact with "modern" people, saw the
world in a more pictorial way than do modern people.
They felt the presence of the gods, their ancestors, and the
spiritual world in general in their daily lives. They thought
more about the health and wellbeing of their group or
tribe and less about their own personal lot in life. Over
the eons, this consciousness has gradually evolved into the
modern human being who conceives of himself as alone in
a universe that is composed only of material "stuff." Or, at
least, there are some who attempt to convince us that this
is the world we live in.

Children, the subject of this book, in their life history,
recapitulate this story of the evolution of humankind. They
start life in a dreamy state in which it is likely they have very
little conception of the things in their lives as distinct, separate entities. They have no names for the items in their lives;
they live entirely in the felt moment—joy with the feeling
of a full tummy, distress when they can't feel the presence

of mom or dad in their world. Out of this dreamy, undifferentiated, feeling state, they gradually evolve, step by step, into the world of walking, talking, and naming the things in their environment, understanding the flow of time and that mom hasn't perished forever if she is out of sight. Musically they flow from the pentatonic scale, as mirrored in their physical body with its four "sets" of five teeth, to the adult octave scale, again mirrored by the four sets of eight teeth in the mouth of the adult. The child grows and evolves all the time, becoming increasingly aware of the reality "out there" and the difference between their inner world and the outer world, between their individual being and the world at large. When all goes well, by the time they are eighteen to twenty-one years old, they are fully developed adults, complete with the modern capacity to picture and understand the world around them and to have some sense of their individuality and their unique place in this larger world. In our time, generally speaking, they have adopted the materialistic "modern" conception of the world, one in which the "gods," "ancestors," and the larger "spiritual world" have become almost, if not completely, obscured.

Their next job, the next journey, as virtually all the modern physicists have pointed out, is to clearly see and understand and even to feel in themselves that this materialistic conception of the world they have evolved into is itself just a step in the process and that, fundamentally, it is an illusion. The journey of life is the fulfillment of our unique destiny and the growing understanding of the spiritual nature of the universe in which we all reside. At its core, the path and suggestions I laid out in this book are meant to help you guide your child "downward" in the descent into materialism, but also to set the stage for the subsequent "ascent" into the next step in human consciousness, which is the felt awareness, the certainty that we are spiritual beings assuming a physical existence as we assume our role in the evolution of our planet and humankind.

Interestingly, when read properly, this is precisely the tale that many of our common fairy tales, the very stories we have told our young children for centuries, are telling. Consider the wonderful and well-known story of Hansel and Gretel. In this tale, two young children are enticed into the forest (always the symbol of the "spiritual world" in fairy tales), where they meet a witch who appears to be suffering from some acute liver disease, with her "yellow eyes," living in a "gingerbread house." My reading of the gingerbread house metaphor is that as we grow up and the spiritual world begins to recede from our awareness, we are inevitably confronted by the phenomenon of materialism as represented by the witch. Although this is inevitable, the sickness of the witch reminds us from the beginning that, if carried too far, this will become a source of sickness for us. As children (but children of all ages for those who never grow up), we are enticed by materialistic "baubles." The gingerbread house in which the witch resides and that enticed Hansel and Gretel is not made of grass-fed kefir, properly soaked oatmeal, biodynamic carrots, or pastured eggs. It is made of counterfeit, empty, poison food—i.e., candy. But, well, it looks good, sort of tastes good, so they are "bewitched," so to speak. This is similar to our modern culture whose people are bewitched into not just accepting but craving and adamantly arguing for their "right" to have fake food, to use chemicals to grow their food instead of compost, to see the fake animals of Disney World instead of experiencing real animals in the woods, who demand the glitzy baubles of fake entertainment on their devices instead of singing in a choir in their church or with their family, and on and on. As Derrick Jensen points out in the title of his book, we are "the culture of make believe," just as the gingerbread house is the dwelling of the diseased witch; it looks bright and shiny, it entices the senses, but it makes you sick down to your core.

Hansel and Gretel, like all of us, can't help but enter this domain, even though they do so initially with trepidation. Upon entering, they find themselves soon shut in a cage, trapped by the cunning and sickness of the witch. Interestingly, if one finds centuries-old drawings depicting these timeless fairy tales, one sees that the cage that the witch puts Hansel and Gretel in has horizontal bars, not the usual vertical bars one would expect. One explanation of this is that these artists, who clearly knew what they were drawing, were showing us that entrapment by the witch primarily entraps the children in the rib cage area (the horizontally shaped ribs), or, in other words, entraps their heart. As I explained in my book *Human Heart, Cosmic Heart*, the human heart is the organ that is the seed of the new "spiritual consciousness" that humans are awakening to. This is precisely the part of the human being the witch is attempting to entrap.

Luckily, the story of Hansel and Gretel provides us the way out of the disease of materialism and a life dominated by baubles instead of real contact with the natural world. In order to extricate himself and Gretel from the cage of materialism and phoniness, Hansel uses two principles that I would suggest are the foundations for humanity's next steps. The first is that Hansel uses his powers of thinking in an imaginative way to present the witch with a chicken bone instead of his finger when the witch is testing his ripeness for eating. The witch, of course, doesn't see properly, just as materialistic science, education, agriculture, and so on also don't see the world properly. Because of this, if we can begin to think clearly about our dilemma, we can find our way out.

The second principle that Hansel uses is his deep devotion to saving not only himself but his sister, Gretel, as well. In other words, the love and caring for the other. When the brother and sister can work together, when they can bring a clear-headed, thoughtful conception of what needs to be done, and merge this with their love and caring for each other, then, and only then, can they find the way out of the forest of despair and materialism. This tale can serve as our model for the answer to the question of how to raise healthy children in a toxic world. Our world is a large gingerbread house. It is full of shiny baubles, which are literally killing us. It is full of make-believe stuff—food, animals, music, and so on.

No matter where you start, no matter your economic situation, no matter how much our society is on the brink of collapse, if you change your mind, magic will happen. The first step is to see your children in a new way. They are unique spiritual beings with strengths, weaknesses, and individual destinies. You are here to help them fulfill this mission. Then you start to put reality in the place of the baubles. Instead of playing them recorded music, sing or tell them stories. Instead of fake food, in all its guises, give them a biodynamically grown raisin, carrot, or pat of butter. Instead of preventing them from going through natural illnesses by using vaccines, Tylenol, and antibiotics, hold them while the fever runs its course. Instead of showing them Disney movies of ridiculous, phony, talking animals, go to a local park and watch the squirrels climb the trees. You take it one step at a time, from whatever place you are starting. You will learn more skills, you will know how to make apple sauce from gleaned apples, saving you money from buying apple sauce at the store. You can learn to mend your own one special pair of socks, saving you money on the continual repurchase of socks you don't even like. If your children are going to school because that is the only option available to you at this point, you make time after school or on the weekends to take a walk in the woods, to visit a farm, to join a choir, to frolic on the beach, to tell each other jokes, to demonstrate the love and care that ultimately saved Hansel and Gretel.

Some may only be in a position to make one small change, such as telling your child stories from your own childhood instead of having them watch a Disney movie. Others will create an unschooled, wireless, no-electronic-devices, complete permaculture type of existence for their family. I welcome both of these and everyone in the middle. For I have seen, in my own life, and in the lives of those around me, that when we dare to take a step, this "spiritual world" will take note and give us a hand. Your children will be grateful for your effort their entire lives.

CHAPTER SIXTEEN

Vaccines and Animals

As we come to the end of this book, it would be good to remind ourselves that the first and most important principle is the admonition to "get on your child's side, and stay there, no matter what." If there is one message I want all my readers to take away it is this simple dictum. But what does it mean in real life to be on your child's side, what does this look like in clear, down-to-earth terms? In this final chapter, I would like to suggest both a positive and "negative" example of what being on your child's side looks like in your life. There are, of course, many other examples of this, but these two examples stand out for me as a kind of litmus test of whether a parent takes this simple admonition to heart, so much so that, no matter what, they cannot be swayed.

The first is the "negative" example, meaning this is not something one does with one's child but rather something that one prevents from being done to your child. That is, any parent, guardian, care-taker or person otherwise responsible for decisions regarding a child in their care will do whatever is necessary to ensure that no children in their care are ever given any so-called vaccine or immunization or any other "preventative" pharmaceutical product for any reason in their life. Again, this book is not meant to be an in-depth scientific explanation for the rationale behind this admonition, for that I have given countless talks, webinars and there are many clear and succinct books that go over this topic in depth. The only point I wish to emphasize here is that unlike some who hope for safer, better tolerated, or more effective vaccines, the real issue with vaccines is that at this point in the history of science and medicine no virus has ever been shown to exist, let alone cause disease, and every trial done in the attempt to prove that bacteria are able to cause disease in well people has failed.

This means the so-called germ theory of disease, as already stated, should be reclassified as the disproven hypothesis that viruses and bacteria are the causative agent of illness in people, animals, or plants. It might help those who are taken aback by this statement to go over the simple case of how a viral vaccine, for example the measles vaccine, is produced. Interestingly, and I encourage all my readers to do this on their own, if you ask your pediatrician or family doctor to explain to you all the steps that go into the production of the measles vaccines, 99% of them will have no clue how this or any vaccine is made. Nor will they be able to tell you how a virus is shown to exist, or even the ingredients in a vaccine. Would you go to a car mechanic because you hear a loud sound whenever you attempt to stop your vehicle only to find out your mechanic has no clue as to the make up or function of a brake?

Let's walk through the basic steps of how a virus is shown to exist and how a live viral vaccine, such as the measles vaccine, is made. Hopefully, once you understand the bizarre, irrational and anti-scientific nature of the procedure you will never waver in your commitment to never allow anyone to give your child any sort of vaccine ever in their life. The first step is they took a child who is said to clinically have measles and removed some mucus from their upper airways. Understand here that even according to the CDC there are many other clinical situations that present with the exact same symptoms as measles, so there is, in fact, no way to know that this child has any specific illness called measles. At this point, you would have no way of knowing the cause of the illness as the alleged viruses cannot be seen by any observer. In the next step, the mucus is filtered to remove any bacteria or cellular debris, so what is left is anything soluble in the mucus of the child. This could include proteins, minerals, other chemicals, toxins, viruses if they existed, or many other things. No attempt at this point is made to identify any virus in the mucus. Then this filtered goop is spread (inoculated) onto a growing culture of highly inbred cells derived from the kidneys of African green monkeys. To this culture is added at least two toxic antibiotics that are known to be specifically toxic to kidney cells, the serum sucked out from a newborn calf's heart, many chemicals such as the enzyme digesting protein called trypsin, and then the nutrient bath that has been keeping the cells alive is diminished. In other words, the growing kidney cells are starved and poisoned and many different substances are added to this culture brew. Then, and this is the key to understanding the entire pseudo-scientific field of virology, if the kidney cells start to die—a process called the cytopathic effect (CPE)—this is taken by *all* virologists to mean that they have identified a virus in the original mucus of the child, and this virus has now been isolated in this process and this is the proof that the virus is the agent that killed the kidney cells. You have got to be kidding!

Interestingly, they stick to this conclusion even though there have been at least five different studies published in the past sixty years, including one that I helped fund in the past four years, that clearly showed that if you repeat all these steps but without adding anything from anyone with measles you get an identical result. This cell culture process, in a use of language that would make Orwell proud, is called the isolation (meaning the separation of one thing from all other things) of the virus, it is the sole proof that the virus exists. Without the isolation of a physical entity, one can't possibly study what it alone is made of or what it alone does. To this there are no exceptions. Therefore, the only possible conclusion one can arrive at is that in spite of hundreds of billions of dollars spent and countless human time spent on virology, they have failed to show any evidence that the thing they are studying even exists.

The important point for this book is that the above broken-down cell culture with all the fetal bovine serum, antibiotic residues, toxic chemicals, is cleaned up a bit and put into vials to be called a "live" viral vaccine, i.e., a measles vaccine. Again, at no point in this procedure was any virus identified, let alone shown to be "alive" or able to cause disease. An attenuated viral vaccine is one in which some of the proteins from this toxic brew have been extracted and put into vials, and an mRNA viral vaccine is one in which some of the RNA from the imaginary, never seen virus has been put into protective coatings and these are put into vials and called vaccines. The bottom line is the injection of this stuff into a living being can only result in a negative outcome, there is no possibility of reward, there is no possibility of this being a road toward health, there is no role for the injection of any such product if the goal is to raise a healthy child.

My hope is that everyone reading this book will make the firm commitment that no matter the obstacles, no matter who pressures you, who attempts to prevent your child from traveling, playing on this or that team, going to this dance class, no matter what, the issue of injecting your child with any pharmaceutical "preventative" medicine is non-negotiable, simply a firm NO. This no is the concrete demonstration of what it means to be on your child's side, no matter what.

The "positive" step that I would suggest is that if there is any way of doing this, I would facilitate every child to have some intimate connection with an animal as they grow up. This is not something that I had much experience with or thought much about as I had never had an emotional connection with an animal until we moved to a homestead in upstate New York and got two kittens to live in the sheep barn next to the sheep and chickens. My thought was that the cats would live in the barn and keep the barn mostly mouse free. Pumpkin had other ideas. After almost every feeding, Pumpkin, our orange male cat, would crawl around my legs until I held him and then sat with him in the garden. Eventually he found his way into the house, onto our bed and into our hearts.

Now, having lived with animals for four years (presently goats, instead of sheep) and having seen children bond with animals, I can say without reservation that a child learning to share life with animals, care for animals, experience the grace, beauty, and passion that animals show for life is perhaps the best way for a child to learn to navigate the world. I have come to understand that when we bring an animal into our lives it is our sacred duty to provide that animal with the means to the best possible life they can have. This means different things for different animals, goats need to roam and eat leaves, cats need to roam freely outside, dogs need to be by their person's side for much of the day, and so on. Our animal guides also need the best food, appropriate to their species, a safe and loving home, and no vaccines, ever. For those who can navigate these parameters, bringing animals into your child's life is a clear way to fulfill the principle of getting on your child's side. Share the care of the animal with your child, be with the animal, talk to your animal. Your child's life will be enriched probably more than any other intervention you can imagine. Animals teach us about the beauty and magical quality of this process called life. Children need to see this beauty; they need to be immersed on a daily basis with the beauty and majesty of this process of life. Your family, connected to all of nature, will teach your child of this mystery, this beauty, this is the final secret of how to raise a healthy child in a toxic world. Let nature, with its crystals, plants, and animals be your guide.

Appendices

1. ELECTROMAGNETIC FREQUENCIES

O n September 28, 2017, a Swedish neuroscientist named Olle Johansson gave a talk on the occasion of the The Madrid International Scientific Declaration on Electromagnetic Fields and Health Effects.* His subject was the effects of EMF fields on biological life and, in particular, what he has discovered after a lifetime of research in this field. The following is a brief synopsis of the main points of his enlightening and sobering lecture. (A video recording of the talk was at one time available on YouTube, and may perhaps appear again.)

The first point he made was that electromagnetic fields were introduced to the world in the late 1800s. Even at that time, some were sounding warnings that this type of energy-generation could and would have negative consequences for living being. As time went on, the EMF fields were intensified and the warnings and findings about the negative effects of these fields, particularly on the growth and development of the children, became more pronounced. If we fast-forward to the twenty-first century, we discover that approximately 25,000 papers have been filed in the peer-reviewed

---

*   A PDF file of the Declaration is available at this URL (accessed May 2024): https://ehtrust.org/wp-content/uploads/Madrid-International -Scientific-Declaration-with-attached-documents-1.pdf.

literature documenting the negative consequences of exposure to modern EMFs.

The World Health Organization (WHO) has classified
routine, current EMF exposure as a probable carcinogen,
in particular linking exposure to EMFs with childhood leukemia. The Council of Europe, upon reviewing the relevant
world literature on the biological consequences of EMFs, has
stated that wireless networks and wireless devices should
be banned from all of the classrooms in Europe and that
this matter is urgent. Furthermore, in a statement released
in 2011, the WHO has stated that routine, current EMF
exposure carries the same risks as exposure to such known
environmental toxins as DDT, lead, welding fumes, formal-
dehyde, and diesel exhaust. They claim that having a child
for six or more hours per day in a classroom with the usual
EMF/wireless exposure subjects them to a risk of "astronom-
ical," "colossal," or "biblical" proportions.

Johansson then went through some of the various relevant
studies done by himself or fellow researchers that document
the specific toxicity to human beings from routine and current EMF levels. For example, when people are exposed to
an electronic device such as a television or computer screen
for one minute, they show increased mast cells in their skin
cells and elevated histamine levels in the skin tissue. These
are the hallmarks of an allergic reaction and exactly the same
reaction one finds upon exposure to medical X-rays.

The next experiment involved normal, healthy Swedish
college students who were asked to sit twenty cm away from
a screen, either a computer or TV while it was on, for one
hour. During and after the exposure, the subjects reported
no symptoms of any kind, but their skin cells showed the

characteristic damage from elevated mast (allergy) cells and the hallmark of elevated histamine levels in their tissues. These findings have been replicated and published in the peer-reviewed literature. The conclusion of the researchers was that exposure to computer screens or TV screens is similar in scope and in damage to that seen with exposure to medical X-rays or uranium.

The next study involved Japanese researchers investigating the effects of exposure to cell phones and their effects on the skin. They found that routine exposure to cell phones increased all the physiological hallmarks of eczema, including elevated levels of substance P, increased polypeptide levels in the skin associated with eczema, and elevated mast cell levels in the skin. They found that the levels of these abnormal findings were directly correlated with the length and severity of the exposure to the cell phone.

Dr. Johansson spoke at length about the known deterioration of the quality of the semen following routine and current EMF exposure. In all cases, with all the studies, semen quality drops upon exposure to EMFs. This drop includes the motility of the sperm, the quantity of the sperm, and the morphology of the sperm. When he presented this and other relevant research to the Minister of Health in Italy, the minister predicted that if this trend continues, the last Italian baby will be conceived around the year 2050. And this is at EMF exposure levels of 2006, not the much higher levels currently in use. With mice studies, they found that even though mice are known to be extraordinarily resistant to damage from EMF exposure, the common, current exposure to EMF fields from the average cell phone or tablet creates widespread infertility, but not until the fifth subsequent generation. In other words, exposure to you now may lead to infertility in your descendants after four or five generations. These warnings should be seen in the context of the dramatic drop in fertility currently being experienced by people all over the Western world.

Routine testing of parameters of heart function and stress levels in newborns and very young children in all cases show deterioration of heart function from exposure to all of the EMF devices currently in use to monitor or teach children. One of the most prominent EMF researchers, Dr. Henry Lye, has shown that rats exposed to routine levels of EMFs show decreased concentration and ability to learn. In particular, their short-term memories seem to be adversely affected by EMF exposure. In a double-blind study he conducted, young boys showed widespread, global reduction in ability to learn new tasks when exposed to minimal, routine EMFs. And along these same lines, a German study showed that one minute of exposure to a cell phone produced demonstrable changes in the EEG (brainwave patterns) for up to one hour after the exposure.

A number of studies confirm the WHO conclusion that routine and current exposure to EMFs is carcinogenic. This includes Spanish studies that show clustering of cancer cases in areas of more intense EMF exposure. This also includes studies showing damage to the DNA occurring in as soon as two hours following exposure to currently available cell phones. A further study likened the exposure that a child would get from being in a class equipped with Wi-Fi for one year to being exposed to 1,600 routine chest X-rays, a level no one would consider acceptable.

In sum, Dr. Johansson has concluded that our current EMF exposure is the largest experiment ever done on living beings. We all have the 24-hour-per-day, 365-day-per-year exposure to a biological toxin on par with DDT, lead, and the other well-known environmental poisons.

He reminds us that the precautionary principle is still the guiding principle of the United Nations and the WHO charters. This means that when there is sufficient suspicion of harm, we should *always* err on the side of caution. This principle is currently being ignored on a level perhaps unseen in human history.

Interestingly, he finishes by relating his experiences when he confronted representatives of the telecom industries or the leaders of the companies who make most of these electronic devices. He says they are well aware of the problem and actually don't dispute the science proving the harm their devices cause. Their only concern is how to avoid liability from the damages that their products cause. Their current solution, one that is in every agreement each of us sign when we purchase an electronic device, is that we are told *never* to allow the device to come within one inch of any part of your body. If you ever touch your cell phone, plug it in your ear, strap it to your wrist, or push the restart button, you have violated the agreement, and the manufacturer is no longer liable for any damages. My guess is they learned how to write these types of agreements in a school, probably law school.

2. TYLENOL

When I was in medical school doing my clinical rotations, I saw two young people who died as a result of a Tylenol overdose. Both were suicides, both took about thirty tablets of regular strength Tylenol and both were brought to the ER too late for their stomachs to be "pumped" or for them to be given charcoal to prevent the absorption of the Tylenol. Once the Tylenol got absorbed into the bloodstream, it was too late and over the next few days they gradually slipped into a hepatic coma and died as a result of liver failure. These are unforgettable experiences for a young doctor and made me wonder about the widespread use of Tylenol for our young children.

Over the years as an ER doctor, it was generally common practice to give children with any amount of temperature elevation a dose of Tylenol, even as they waited in the waiting room to be seen by the physician. That's how safe Tylenol is considered to be, even for the very youngest children. There is a tendency in our culture to use one's lengthy experience with some substance or some task as evidence that the person involved is somehow an expert in that particular subject. Sometimes, it holds true. A car mechanic who has fixed one thousand Volvos is likely to be an expert in Volvo mechanics. On the other hand, having eaten one thousand bags of potato chips doesn't make someone an expert in the harmful effect of a junk-food diet. Similarly, just because a pediatrician has given over a thousand doses of Tylenol, it doesn't prove they are expert in Tylenol toxicity. The reality is it's likely they know nothing about the subject at all.

Tylenol has two major problems, which combined make it an unsafe, unfit medicine to use with any child, no matter the situation. The first problem, which I covered extensively in my vaccine book, is that fever is the body's primary mechanism for overcoming any type of toxin condition. As Hippocrates said, "Give me a medicine to produce a fever and I can cure any disease." Fevers themselves, no matter the height of the temperature, do not damage the child in any way. They can be a sign that something is wrong. A child with meningitis, for example, is in grave danger and the fever is one of the ways the body alerts us that something is wrong. But we must be very clear that it's the toxic condition in the brain that kills the child, the fever is the body's way of fighting back. It makes no sense, none at all, to use Tylenol or any other pharmaceutical medicine to bring down a fever. The medical literature is absolutely clear on this issue—artificially reducing the temperature in an acutely ill child prolongs the illness and makes complications, such as pneumonia, "ear infections," etc., more likely to occur. Children with the condition referred to as measles who use Tylenol have worse outcomes than children whose caregivers let the fever take its course. There is no medical indication for bringing down a fever with pharmaceuticals, none. Every pediatrician knows this, or at least should know it, even though they pretend they don't. By bringing the fever down with Tylenol, you are doing the child a huge disservice.

Clearly, I am not saying a child with a fever is not sick or that in unusual situations some bad outcome could never happen. Children with fevers should be observed in order to understand the severity of the underlying illness. They can be given natural medicines like liposomal vitamin C every hour while awake to help them detoxify. Liposomal vitamin C and many other natural medicines can and should be used with febrile illnesses. None of them are meant to lower the fever—no natural medicine can or should do that. That is the arsenal we use to heal.

The second and mostly ignored and unrecognized problem with Tylenol is that the research is suggesting that Tylenol is a potent neurotoxic substance that has many widespread deleterious effects on the brain of the growing child. This first study looked at the use of Tylenol in pregnancy and its effect on the neurological development of the growing child. Here is the conclusion of the article:

> Children exposed to acetaminophen prenatally are at increased risk of multiple behavioral difficulties, and the associations do not appear to be explained by unmeasured behavioral or social factors linked to acetaminophen use insofar as they are not observed for postnatal or partner's acetaminophen use. Although these results could have implications for public health advice, further studies are required to replicate the findings and to understand mechanisms.*

As always, the conclusions are couched in cautious medical speak, but their research is suggesting that Tylenol use in pregnancy is an independent factor associated with behavioral problems later for the child.

---

*   "Association of Acetaminophen Use During Pregnancy with Behavioral Problems in Childhood Evidence Against Confounding." Evie Stergiakouli, PhD1; Anita Thapar, FRCPsych, PhD2; George Davey Smith, MD, DSc. *JAMA Pediatr.* 2016; 170(10): 964-970. doi:10.1001/jamapediatrics.2016.1775.

This next study, also in a peer-reviewed medical journal, documents the relationship between prenatal Tylenol use and the later diagnosis of autism in the child:

Conclusions: Prenatal acetaminophen exposure was associated with a greater number of autism-spectrum symptoms in males and showed adverse effects on attention-related outcomes for both genders. These associations seem to be dependent on the frequency of exposure.*

Their findings were particularly interesting because they were able to show that Tylenol is more toxic to the brains of male children than female children and that, as one might expect from a problem caused by a toxic exposure, the greater the exposure, the higher the toxicity.

An excerpt from the conclusion of the next peer-reviewed study also correlates the autism epidemic to the increased and widespread use of Tylenol. Here is their conclusion:

Acetaminophen (paracetamol) is a widely used over-the-counter (OTC) analgesic and antipyretic that was introduced since 1955 [3]. Unfortunately, the recent mechanistic evidence suggests correlation between acet-aminophen exposure and increased incidence and risk of autism [4–6]. Considerable evidence supports this contention, most notably the exponential chronologi-cal rise in acetaminophen consumption for infants and young children since the 1980s when it began to replace

---

* "Acetaminophen Use in Pregnancy and Neurodevelopment: Attention Function and Autism Spectrum Symptoms." Claudia B. Avella-Garcia, Jordi Julvez, Joan Fortuny, Cristina Rebordosa, Raquel García-Esteban, Isolina Riaño, Galán Adonina Tardón, Clara L. Rodríguez-Bernal, Carmen Iñiguez, Ainara Andiarena. *International Journal of Epidemiology*, Volume 45, Issue 6, 1 Dec. 2016, pp. 1,987–1,996; https://doi.org/10.1093/ije/dyw115.

aspirin [7]. For instance, this compound has been taken, at least once, by more than 85% of children under the age of 91 months in the UK [8]. Children who are poor metabolizers of acetaminophen may be at higher risk even under therapeutic doses [5].*

This is not to suggest that Tylenol use is the sole cause of autism—it's clearly not—but it does show and suggest that Tylenol is a neurotoxin and therefore cannot be safely used by any young child.

These next two studies also conclude that prenatal exposure to Tylenol has adverse consequences for higher neurological function in the children. This includes the acquisition of social skills and the development of empathy:

> These findings strengthen the contention that acetaminophen exposure in pregnancy increases the risk of ADHD-like behaviors. Our study also supports earlier claims that findings are specific to acetaminophen.**
>
> Conclusions: We found some evidence that maternal paracetamol use during pregnancy was associated with poorer attention and executive function in five-year-olds.***

----

* Acetaminophen/Autism: Alarm? Amany A. Abdin (2013), *Biochem Pharmacol* (Los Angel) 2:e148. doi:10.4172/2167-0501.1000e148.

** "Associations between Acetaminophen Use during Pregnancy and ADHD Symptoms Measured at Ages 7 and 11 Years." Thompson JM1, Waldie KE2, Wall CR3, Murphy R4, Mitchell EA1; ABC Study Group. *PLOS One*. Sept. 24, 2014; 9(9):e108210. doi: 10.1371/journal.pone.0108210. eCollection 2014.

*** "Paracetamol Use during Pregnancy and Attention and Executive Function in Offspring at Age 5 years." Zeyan Liew, Catherine Carlsen Bach, Robert F. Asarnow, Beate Ritz, Jørn Olsen. *International Journal of Epidemiology*, Volume 45, Issue 6, Dec. 1, 2016, pp. 2,009–2,017; https://doi.org/10.1093/ije/dyw296. Published: December 29, 2016.

Again, these are studies published in peer-reviewed medical journals that should alert us to the neurotoxic effects of Tylenol. The precautionary principle in medicine, that toxic substances should not be used until they are proven to be safe, a principle codified in the WHO and UN charters, are clearly being blatantly ignored by the widespread use of Tylenol in our current pediatric clinics.

Tylenol use in large amounts, all at once, kills people from liver damage. The routine use of Tylenol for acute, febrile illness prolongs their suffering and makes them have a higher likelihood of a poor outcome from their illness. Tylenol appears to be a potent neurotoxic substance and is associated with damage to higher functions in the brains of young children. Given these clear facts, tell me again why we are using millions and millions of doses per year on our young children and pregnant mothers?

3. Diagnostic Ultrasounds

A lmost 100 percent of pregnant women in the U.S. have at least one diagnostic ultrasound (DUS) during pregnancy. Like X-rays and exposure to EMFs, when asked if DUS is safe in pregnancy, most respond that they don't feel anything unusual during the ultrasound and the medical authorities tell us they are safe, so they must be safe. By now, we probably realize that neither of these responses are reassuring. Ultrasound technology is an offshoot of Sonar technology developed originally for military uses. It basically involves bouncing a high frequency, unnatural beam of energy at an object and measuring the time it takes for an image to "bounce back." The frequencies involved are higher than the usual EMF frequencies and about a thousand times higher than the pain threshold for the human ear. In pregnancy, they are used to assess the status of the fetus, define the anatomy of the fetus, to check dates and progress of the fetus, or to just get a nice picture of the fetus.

In 1982, the WHO sounded the original alarm about the dangers of DUS when they stated that the cavitations and "bubbles" produced by the powerful sound waves of DUS could have adverse health consequences for the developing fetus.* Soon afterward, there were growing reports

---

*   "Environmental Health Criteria 22: Ultrasound," published by the World Health Organization, 1982.

of mothers claiming a variety of untoward experiences in the immediate aftermath of DUS. These symptoms include change in the movement of the fetus during and following the procedure, maternal pain during and following the procedure, and occasional vaginal bleeding during and after the procedure. Around this time, many research labs were starting to publish their findings on the dangers of DUS for laboratory animals. Here is the conclusion of one such study done by the Bioacoustics Research Laboratory at the University of Illinois:

> More than thirty-five published animal studies suggest that in utero ultrasound exposure can affect prenatal growth.... A number of biological effects have been observed following ultrasound exposure in various experimental systems. These include reduction in immune response, change in sister chromatid exchange frequencies, cell death, change in cell membrane functions, degradation of macromolecules, free radical formation, and reduced cell reproductive potential.... The data on clinical efficacy and safety do not allow a recommendation for routine screening.*

In other words, no matter what biological parameter they chose to measure, they found convincing evidence that DUS was unsafe for the developing fetus.

The next significant study was done in 1993 by a researcher named Newnham, who tested the safety of DUS using ultrasound machines that are at least ten times *less* intense than those currently approved for use. Here is his conclusion: "Our findings suggested that (five or more ultrasound sessions) increase the proportion of growth-restricted

---

*   Ibid.

fetuses by about one third.... It would seem prudent to limit ultrasound examination of the fetus."*

As time went on, human studies started to be done. One done by Stalberg in 2008 came to this conclusion: "Boys exposed to ultrasound at any time during gestation had lower mean grades in physical education and a tendency toward lower school grades in general."**

It's not that I have suddenly changed my mind about school, but I'm not sure we want to do a medical procedure on our children that makes them less coordinated and less "intelligent."

DUS has long been recognized to be problematic for one's eyes due to its tendency to produce bubbles and cavitations in fluids because of its heating effect. Since 1980, the FDA has set the limits for exposure of the adult eye at an intensity of 50 mW/cm2. The current DUS level used in the examination of the fetus is set at 720 mW/cm2. There is no attempt made in our current DUS examination of the fetus to shield the eyes of the fetus from this current exposure, even though it should be clear to all that the fetal eyes are more exposed and more sensitive than those of adults.

More recent studies were done in China in which women who were planning on having abortions were randomized to either receive DUS or not in a blinded experiment. The researchers measured damage to the fetal tissues as a consequence of the DUS exposure. Their conclusions were that

---

*   Newnham, J. P., et al. "Effects of Frequent Ultrasound during Pregnancy: A Randomised Controlled Trial," *Lancet* 342, no. 8876 (Oct. 9, 1993), pp. 887–891.

**   Stalberg, K., et al., "Multiple Ultrasound Exposure and School Achievement in Teenagers; Follow-up of a Randomised Controlled Trial," *Ultrasound in Obstetrics and Gynecology* 32, no. 3 (2008), pp. 303–306.

low exposure to DUS is "damaging to the human fetus, ovum and embryo, at all time durations of exposure." This included exposures in the seconds, not in the minutes as the DUS is currently performed. They were able to document damage to the fetal DNA due to DUS exposure with implications for the developing immune system of the fetus and for the possible incidence of childhood leukemia.

Finally, very few real safety studies have been done on DUS. One study published in 1992 by D. L. Miller concluded: "The allowable output for obstetrical ultrasound was increased (8x15X).... There has been little or no subsequent research...to systematically assess potential risks to the fetus." *

Sadly, almost thirty years later, the situation hasn't changed much, and still no adequate safety trials have been performed. This situation is sadly reminiscent of the story of vaccines, EMFs, Tylenol, and many other toxic medical interventions. Some "unnatural" medical intervention, one that seems to have great promise, is introduced. For a few, as is the case with DUS, there is valuable information obtained, even information that can save the life of a mother or her child.

Then, somehow, the procedure morphs into something that is used for everyone, with very little evidence that it improves outcomes when widely used or that it is safe in this setting. Then, for some reason, once it becomes an entrenched part of the medical system, the safety trials somehow dry up, and anyone who dares question the safety of this procedure is widely and loudly criticized. The science showing harm is

---

*   Miller D. L. et al. "Overview of Therapeutic Ultrasound Applications and Safety Considerations," *Journal of Ultrasound in Medicine* 31, no. 4 (April 1, 2012), pp. 623–634.

ignored or ridiculed; people begin to say that it must be safe because it's been in use for X number of years. Meanwhile, the children get sicker and sicker, we build multibillion-dollar hospitals devoted to treating children with cancers, seemingly never stopping to ask the fundamental question: How come we have so many sick children? How come so many children have cancer these days?

To be clear, I am not against the use of DUS in cases in which the results of the examination can and will lead to a clear therapeutic intervention that delivers benefit to mother or child. But I am completely against the use of an unsafe examination for any routine pregnancy unless and until this test is conclusively proven to be safe, which in my opinion will never happen.

Bibliography

Booth, Mark. *The Secret History of the World: As Laid Down by the Secret Societies*. Woodstock, NY: Overlook, 2008.

Cowan, Thomas. *Human Heart, Cosmic Heart: A Doctor's Quest to Understand, Treat, and Prevent Cardiovascular Disease*. White River Junction, VT: Chelsea Green, 2016.

———. *Vaccines, Autoimmunity, and the Changing Nature of Childhood Illness*. White River Junction, VT: Chelsea Green, 2018.

Fallon, Sally. *Nourishing Traditions: The Cookbook that Challenges Politically Correct Nutrition and the Diet Dictocrats*. Brandywine, MD: NewTrends, 1999, 2001.

Fallon Morell, Sally, and Thomas S. Cowan. *The Nourishing Traditions Book of Baby and Child Care*. Washington, DC: NewTrends, 2013.

Illich, Ivan. *Deschooling Society*. London/New York: Marion Boyars, 2000.

———. *The Right to Useful Unemployment: And Its Professional Enemies*. London/New York: Marion Boyars, 2000.

Kohn, Alfie. *Punished by Rewards: The Trouble with Gold Stars, Incentive Plans, A's, Praise, and Other Bribes*. Boston/New York: Mariner, 1993, 2018.

Mander, Jerry. *In The Absence of the Sacred: The Failure of Technology and the Survival of the Indian Nations*. Oakland, CA: Sierra Club Books, 1991.

Perlas, Nicanor. *Humanity's Last Stand: The Challenge of Artificial Intelligence: A Spiritual-Scientific Response*. Forest Row, UK: Temple Lodge, 2018.

Steiner, Rudolf. *The Gospel of John*. Spencertown, NY: SteinerBooks, 2022.

———. *The Kingdom of Childhood: Introductory Talks on Waldorf Education*. Hudson, NY: Anthroposophic Press, 1995.

Tucker, Jim B. *Life before Life: A Scientific Investigation of Children's Memories of Previous Lives*. New York: St. Martin's, 2005.

———. *Return to Life: Extraordinary Cases of Children Who Remember Past Lives*. New York: St. Martin's, 2013.

Index

addiction to electronic
  devices, 116–18
Ali, Muhammad,
  14, 45
alternative medicine,
  27
Alternative Therapies,
  27
animal(s)
  care for, 138–39
  intimate bonding
    with, 138–39
  weather-controlled
    domes, 27–28
animal foods, 96
antibiotics, 25–26,
  132, 136

bacteria, 25, 135
battle of wills, 66
Bioacoustics Research
  Laboratory at the
  University
  of Illinois, 153
blank slate theory,
  121, 126
Bohr, Niels, 127
Booth, Mark, 109

canine movement
  specialists, 90
caring, 132
charter schools, 74
child study(ies), 4–5
chronic illness, 25, 50.
  See also diseases/
  illness
Chuang Tzu, 56
Churchill, Winston, 76
climbing, 19–21
clot-busting drug,
  42–43
coercion, 21

college degree, 87–88
Common Sense (Paine),
  81–82, 106
communication, 21–22
compulsory education/
  schooling. *See*
  school/schooling
consciousness, 109–10,
  122, 128, 130
  collective, 126
  congealed, 122
  imitative, 109
  spiritual, 131
consumer society, 38
Council of Europe, 142
Crime and Punishment
  (Dostoyevsky), 73
currency creation,
  114–15
curriculum. *See* hidden
  curriculum
cytopathic effect
  (CPE), 136

democracy, 81–82, 87
Deschooling Society
  (Illich), 73–74,
  78–79
Dewey, John, 76
diagnostic ultrasound
  (DUS), 69, 152–56
diets, 50, 69
  animal foods, 96
  plant foods, 97
  seed foods, 96–97
  traditional, 51,
    96–98
discipline/disciplining
  children
  alternative way to
    approach, 60–70
  avoiding battle of
    wills, 66

engagement, 62
  saying "no," 61–62
  See also punishments
    and rewards
diseases/illness, 25–28
  healing patterns, 26
  immune system and,
    26, 28
  infectious, 28
  See also vaccines
Division of Perceptual
  Studies, University
  of Virginia,
  121–22
Dossey, Larry, 27
Duncan, Arne, 87–88

Eccles, John C., 126
educational culture/
  model
  administrative
    techniques,
    101–2
  cultivating interests
    and individual
    genius, 100–103
  dietary insights,
    96–98
  exposure to special
    interests, 103
  homestead (*see*
    homestead
    work)
  subsistence activities,
    98–99, 103
  tolerance, 93–96
  See also school/
    schooling
educational program,
  120
electromagnetic
  frequencies (EMF),
  113, 141–45

electronic devices,
    115–19
    addiction to, 116–18
    infrastructure,
        115–16
    mitigating influence
        of, 118–19
employment, 37, 90.
    See also work

Fallon, Sally, 96
fear of illiteracy, 106
food
    non-interference with
        consumption
        of, 52
    procurement, 98
    production, 22–23,
        98
    quality, 53
    See also diets
food fights, 50–55
    autonomy and,
        51–53
    Rosenberg on, 51
    solution to, 51
force. See protective
    use of force
Fowles, John, 77–78

Galilei, Galileo, 75
Gatto, John, 81
Genentech, 43, 46
germ theory, 25, 135
Goethe, Johann
    Wolfgang von, 12
The Gospel of St. John
    (Steiner), 73
greeting, 49

hemorrhagic strokes,
    42–43
hidden curriculum,
    74, 79, 83–92.
    See also radical
    monopoly; school/
    schooling
Holt, John, 56, 86, 87
homestead work,

18–19, 98–99, 103
Human Heart, Cosmic
    Heart (Cowan),
    39, 131
Humanity's Last Stand
    (Perlas), 116
humiliation, 47–48.
    See also shame/
    shaming

Illich, Ivan, 37, 101,
    102
    on compulsory
        schooling,
        78–79, 91
    Deschooling Society,
        73–74, 78–79
    radical monopoly,
        83, 85
illiteracy, 106
illness. See diseases/
    illness
immune system, 26, 28
immunization. See
    vaccines
infectious disease, 28
integrity, 42–49
    examples, 42–46
    greeting and, 49
    modeling, 47–48
    stories of, 48–49
In the Absence of the
    Sacred (Manders),
    98
intolerance, 93–94. See
    also tolerance
ischemic strokes, 42

Jensen, Derrick, 131
jobs. See work
Johansson, Olle, 141,
    142, 143, 145

Kearns, David T., 77
Kohn, Alfie, 58, 68

learning
    about tolerance,
        93–95

being taught and,
    86–87
dietary insights,
    96–98
exposure and, 23
natural curiosity, 87
non-coerced
    experience, 23
reading, 106–12
See also educational
    culture/model;
    school/schooling
Life before Life
    (Tucker), 122
love, 12, 132
Lye, Henry, 144

Madrid International
    Scientific
    Declaration on
    Electromagnetic
    Fields and Health
    Effects, 141
mandatory schooling.
    See school/
    schooling
Manders, Jerry, 98
measles
    Tylenol and, 147
    vaccine, 135–36, 137
memories of past lives,
    121–25
Mencken, H. L., 76
mental health, 10, 13
Merck, 44–46
military conscription,
    14
Miller, D. L., 155
The Mists of Avalon,
    109
modeling integrity,
    47–48
money, 36–37, 39, 133
    radical monopoly
        and, 90
    monopolistic behavior,
        83. See also radical
        monopoly
moral judgments,
    13–14

nap, 21. *See also* sleep
natural world, 69–70
Newnham, JP, 153–54
Nietzsche, Friedrich,
75–76, 100
Nokken, Copenhagen,
16–23
non-productive
activities, 104
nonviolent
communication
(NVC), 4
*Nourishing Traditions
Book of Baby and
Child Care, The*
12, 34, 69

oppositional-defiance
disorder, 10, 13

Paine, Thomas, 81
Palin, Sarah, 39
Papert, Seymour, 77
past lives. *See*
memories of past
lives
Penrose, Roger, 126–27
Perlas, Nicanor, 116
perseverance, 24–33
challenges/stressors
and, 24, 28–33
developing strength
through, 24
diseases/illness and,
25–28
PhD graduates, 89–90,
91
plant foods, 97
plants, 27–28
plaque-based
blockages, 42.
See also ischemic
strokes
Plato, 75
play, 34–41, 99
definition, 35
practical and serious
activities, 39–41
public education and,
38

work and, 35–41
"play 60" campaigns,
35
plorking, 38, 40
pneumonia, 25–26
pregnancy, 148, 150,
152
nutrition in, 69
prenatal ultrasounds.
See diagnostic
ultrasound (DUS)
Price, Weston A.,
96–97
protective use of force,
61
Punished by Rewards
(Kohn), 58
punishments and
rewards, 56–68,
75
avoiding battle of
wills, 66
being counter-
productive,
66–68
educators and,
58–59, 60
harms through, 58,
66–68
parents and, 58,
59–60
as self-defeating
concepts, 60

qualities of human
beings, 12–13

racial tension, 29–30,
32
racism, 93
radical monopoly, 120
consequence or
example of,
83–85
defined, 83
government/
corporate
conglomerate,
90
money and, 90

schooling, 85–92,
104
reading, 106–12
consciousness,
109–10
Steiner on, 106–8
restorative justice,
46–47
Return to Life (Tucker),
122
rewards. *See*
punishments and
rewards
*The Right to Useful
Unemployment*
(Illich), 37
Rogers, Carl, 5
Rosenberg, Marshall,
5, 58

schooled society, 87
school/schooling,
73–82
Churchill on, 76
coerced, 96
core idea of, 87
Dewey on, 76
Duncan on, 87–88
educational
guidelines and,
80
Fowles on, 77–78
fundamental
premises of,
80–81
Galilei on, 75
hidden curriculum,
74, 79, 83–92
Illich on, 78–79, 91
Kearns on, 77
Mencken on, 76
Nietzsche on, 75–76
Papert on, 77
Plato on, 75
racial tension, 29–30
radical monopolies,
85–92, 104
Twain on, 77, 80
universal, 74
Wilde on, 76

Secret History of the World, The (Booth), 109
seed foods, 96–97
segregation, 30
self-sufficiency, 17
settled science, 113–14
shame/shaming, 47–48
sleep, 98. *See also* nap
social media, 117
spiritual consciousness, 131
splinter. *See* diseases/illness
Stalberg, K., 154
Steiner, Rudolf, 12, 110, 111, 112, 119
  educational philosophy, 109
  The Gospel of St. John, 73
  law of reincarnation, 126
  on learning to read, 106–8
  pedagogy, 109
Stevenson, Ian, 121
storytelling, 21–22
stressors, 24, 28–33
strokes
  clot-busting drugs for, 42–43
  hemorrhagic, 42
  ischemic, 42–43
subsistence activities, 98–99, 103. *See also* homestead work
suffering, 47
sugar foods, 50
Sullivan, Anne, 58–59

Swaziland, 73, 98–99
  confiscation of property, 84
  extended family, 54
  food/meals/diets, 54–55, 97
  radical monopoly and, 83–84

telling stories. *See* storytelling
To Kill a Mockingbird, 48
tolerance, 93–96
  mandatory course, 94–95
toxic antibiotics, 136
traditional diets, 51, 96–98
traumatic experience, 125
tree climbing. *See* climbing
trust, 12–15
trypsin, 136
Tucker, Jim, 122
Twain, Mark, 14, 77, 80
Tylenol, 146–51

ultrasound technology, 152–156
Underground History of American Education, The (Gatto), 81

vaccines, 43–44, 134–38
Vaccines, Autoimmunity, and the Changing Nature of Childhood Illness, 12
Vietnam, 14
violence
  protective use of force, 61
  shame/humiliation inflicting, 47
Vioxx, 44–45
viral vaccine, 137–38
viruses, 135–137
  as an imaginary construct, 26

wage-slaves, 39
Waldorf schools, 4–9, 62, 105, 108–12
weather-controlled domes, 27–28
"Weather Deficiency Syndrome" (Dossey), 27
Weston A. Price Foundation, 102
Wilde, Oscar, 76
work, 98
  access to money, 36–37
  definition, 35
  misery, 37
  play and, 35–41
  public education and, 38
World Health Organization (WHO), 142, 144, 151
  on dangers of DUS, 152